AF587981

PHARMACOLOGY – RESEARCH, SAFETY TESTING AND REGULATION SERIES

SAFETY EFFORTS IN PEDIATRIC DRUG DEVELOPMENT

Pharmacology – Research, Safety Testing and Regulation Series

Antibiotic Resistance: Causes and Risk Factors, Mechanisms and Alternatives
Adriel R. Bonilla and Kaden P. Muniz (Editors)
2009. ISBN: 978-1-60741-623-4

Antibiotic Resistance: Causes and Risk Factors, Mechanisms and Alternatives
Adriel R. Bonilla and Kaden P. Muniz (Editors)
2009. ISBN: 978-1-61668-162-3 (Online Book)

Poisons: Physiologically Active Substances
S. B. Zotov and O. I. Tuzhikov
2009. ISBN: 978-1-60741-973-0

Drug Monitoring by HPLC: Recent Developments
Victoria Samanidou and Eftichia Karageorgou
2010. ISBN: 978-1-60876-183-8

Nonprescription Drugs: Considering A New Class for Behind-the-Counter Drugs
Lars P. Eliassen (Editor)
2010. ISBN: 978-1-60741-961-7

Biogenic Amines: Pharmacological, Neurochemical, and Molecular Aspects in the CNS
Tahira Farooqui and Akhlaq A. Farooqui (Editors)
2010. ISBN: 978-1-60876-625-3

Handbook of Drug Targeting and Monitoring
Boris Andreev and Vasily Egorov (Editors)
2010 ISBN: 978-1-60741-839-9

Biopharmaceutics and Drug Hypersensitivity
Paul Mossillo and John Pinzini (Editors)
2010 ISBN: 978-1-60741-830-6

Multiple Drug Resistance
Agoston Meszaros and Gusztav Balogh (Editors)
2010 ISBN: 978-1-60741-595-4

Safety Efforts in Pediatric Drug Development
Conor D. Byrne (Editor)
2010 ISBN: 978-1-60741-565-7

PHARMACOLOGY – RESEARCH, SAFETY TESTING AND REGULATION SERIES

SAFETY EFFORTS IN PEDIATRIC DRUG DEVELOPMENT

CONOR D. BYRNE
EDITOR

Nova Science Publishers, Inc.
New York

LIBRARY OF CONGRESS CATALOGING-IN-PUBLICATION DATA

Safety efforts in pediatric drug development / [edited by] Conor D. Byrne.
p. ; cm.
Includes index.
ISBN 978-1-60741-565-7 (hardcover)
1. Pediatric pharmacology--United States. 2. Pediatrics--United States--Formulae, receipts, prescriptions--Safety measures. 3. Drug development--United States--Safety measures. 4. United States. Best Pharmaceuticals for Children Act. I. Byrne, Conor D.
[DNLM: 1. United States. Best Pharmaceuticals for Children Act. 2. Drug Approval--United States. 3. Child--United States. 4. Drug Evaluation--standards--United States. 5. Drug Toxicity--prevention & control--United States. 6. Legislation, Drug--United States. QV 771 S1282 2009]
RJ560.S24 2009, 615'.190083--dc22, 2009031817

Published by Nova Science Publishers, Inc. ✦ New York

Chapter Sources

The following chapters have been previously published:

Chapter 1 – This is an edited, excerpted and augmented edition of a United States Congressional Research Service publication, Report Order Code RL33986, dated December 2, 2008.

Chapter 2 – This is an edited, excerpted and augmented edition of a United States Department of Health and Human Services, Food and Drug Administration, Centre for Drug Evaluation and Research (CDER) publication, dated February 2006.

Chapter 3 - This is an edited, excerpted and augmented edition of a United States Government Accountability Office (GAO), Report to Congressional Committees. Publication GAO-07-557, dated March 2007.

Chapter 4 – These remarks were delivered as Statement of Marcia Crosse, Director, Health Care, before the Subcommittee on Health Committee on Energy and Commerce, U.S. House of Representatives, dated May 22, 2007.

Contents

PREFACE

This book focuses on the safety efforts being implemented in pediatric drug development. Although children suffer from many of the same diseases as adults and are often treated with the same drugs, only about one-third of the drugs that are prescribed for children have been studied and labeled for pediatric use. This has placed children taking drugs for which there have not been adequate pediatric drug studies at risk of being exposed to ineffective treatment or receiving incorrect dosing. In order to encourage the study of more drugs for pediatric use, Congress passed the Best Pharmaceuticals for Children Act (BPCA) in 2002 to provide marketing incentives to drug manufacturers for conducting pediatric drug studies. Drug manufacturers may obtain six months of additional market exclusivity for drugs on which they have conducted pediatric studies in accordance with pertinent law and regulations. This book also evaluates the impact of BPCA on labeling drugs for pediatric use and the process by which the labeling was changed, and illustrates the range of diseases treated by the drugs studied under BPCA. Additionally this book provides guidance on the role and timing of animal studies in the nonclinical safety evaluation of therapeutics intended for the treatment of pediatric patients. The guidance discusses some conditions under which juvenile animals can be meaningful predictors of toxicity in pediatric patients and makes recommendations on nonclinical testing.

This book consists of public documents which have been located, gathered, combined, reformatted, and enhanced with a subject index, selectively edited and bound to provide easy access.

Chapter 1 - In 2007 Congress reauthorized two laws allowing the Food and Drug Administration (FDA) to offer financial and regulatory incentives to test their products for use in children. Through the Food and Drug Administration Amendments Act of 2007 (FDAAA, P.L. 110-85), Congress extended both the

Best Pharmaceuticals for Children Act (BPCA) and the Pediatric Research Equity Act (PREA) for five years.

About 75% of drugs have not had pediatric studies. The laws address concerns that clinicians must often prescribe drugs for children that FDA has approved only for adult use. Clinicians often take that step believing that the safety and effectiveness demonstrated with adults would hold for younger patients. But studies show that drugs vary in bioavailability in children, which depends on the maturation and development of organs and other factors. Therefore, this off-label prescribing results in some children's receiving ineffective drugs or too much or too little of a potentially useful drug. It may also result in side effects unique to children, or children of specific ages, including effects on growth and development.

The market has not been able to overcome the economic, ethical, legal, and mechanical obstacles that make manufacturers reluctant to conduct these tests. The reauthorized BPCA and PREA represent ongoing involvement of Congress and FDA to address this need. FDA had tried unsuccessfully to spur pediatric drug research through administrative action before 1997. With the FDA Modernization Act of 1997 (FDAMA, P.L. 105-115), Congress provided an incentive: in exchange for a manufacturer's completion of pediatric studies according to an FDA written request, FDA would extend its market exclusivity for that product for six months. BPCA (P.L. 107-109) gave this program a five-year reauthorization in 2002. To get pediatric use information on the drugs that manufacturers were not studying, in 1998, FDA published the Pediatric Rule requiring that manufacturers submit pediatric testing data at the time of all new drug applications. In 2002, a federal court declared the rule invalid, holding that FDA lacked the statutory authority to promulgate it. Congress gave FDA that authority with PREA (P.L. 108-155). PREA covers drugs and biological products and includes provisions for deferrals, waivers, and the required pediatric assessment of an approved marketed product.

Some of the issues the 110th Congress considered remain of concern. Why offer a financial incentive to encourage pediatric studies when FDA has the authority to require them? How does the cost of marketing exclusivity—including the higher prices paid by government—compare with the cost of the needed research? What percentage of drug labeling includes adequate pediatric information because of BPCA and PREA? Does the law provide FDA with sufficient authority to act and does FDA choose to so act? These kinds of questions—determining what information clinicians and consumers need, how to then develop and disseminate it; how to balance carrots and sticks; and how to consider cost and benefit—could not only help the 111th Congress evaluate BPCA and PREA, but also inform its consideration of healthcare reform.

Chapter 2 - This guidance represents the Food and Drug Administration's (FDA's) current thinking on this topic. It does not create or confer any rights for or on any person and does not operate to bind FDA or the public. You can use an alternative approach if the approach satisfies the requirements of the applicable statutes and regulations. If you want to discuss an alternative approach, contact the FDA staff responsible for implementing this guidance. If you cannot identify the appropriate FDA staff, call the appropriate number listed on the title page of this guidance.

Chapter 3 - About two-thirds of drugs that are prescribed for children have not been studied and labeled for pediatric use, which places children at risk of being exposed to ineffective treatment or incorrect dosing. The Best Pharmaceuticals for Children Act (BPCA), enacted in 2002, encourages the manufacturers, or sponsors, of drugs that still have marketing exclusivity—that is, are on-patent—to conduct pediatric drug studies, as requested by the Food and Drug Administration (FDA). If they do so, FDA may extend for 6 months the period during which no equivalent generic drugs can be marketed. This is referred to as pediatric exclusivity.

BPCA required that GAO assess the effect of BPCA on pediatric drug studies and labeling. As discussed with the committees of jurisdiction, GAO (1) assessed the extent to which pediatric drug studies were being conducted under BPCA for on-patent drugs, including when drug sponsors declined to conduct the studies; (2) evaluated the impact of BPCA on labeling drugs for pediatric use and the process by which the labeling was changed; and (3) illustrated the range of diseases treated by the drugs studied under BPCA. GAO examined data about the drugs for which FDA requested studies under BPCA from 2002 through 2005. GAO also interviewed officials from relevant federal agencies, pharmaceutical industry representatives, and health advocates.

www.gao.gov/cgi-bin/getrpt?GAO-07-557.

To view the full product, including the scope and methodology, click on the link above. For more information, contact Marcia Crosse at (202) 512-7119 or crossem@gao.gov.

Chapter 4 - About two-thirds of drugs that are prescribed for children have not been studied and labeled for pediatric use, placing children at risk of being exposed to ineffective treatment or incorrect dosing. The Best Pharmaceuticals for Children Act (BPCA), enacted in 2002, encourages the manufacturers, or sponsors, of drugs that still have marketing exclusivity—that is, are on-patent—to conduct pediatric drug studies, as requested by the Food and Drug Administration

(FDA). If they do so, FDA may extend for 6 months the period during which no equivalent generic drugs can be marketed. This is referred to as pediatric exclusivity. BPCA also provides for the study of off-patent drugs.

GAO was asked to testify on the study and labeling of drugs for pediatric use under BPCA. This testimony is based on *Pediatric Drug Research: Studies Conducted under Best Pharmaceuticals for Children Act,* GAO-07-557 (Mar. 22, 2007). GAO assessed (1) the extent to which pediatric drug studies were being conducted under BPCA for on-patent drugs, (2) the extent to which pediatric drug studies were being conducted under BPCA for off-patent drugs, and (3) the impact of BPCA on the labeling of drugs for pediatric use and the process by which the labeling was changed. GAO examined data about the drugs for which FDA requested studies under BPCA from 2002 through 2005 and interviewed relevant federal officials.

www.gao.gov/cgi-bin/getrpt?GAO-07-898T.

To view the full product, including the scope and methodology, click on the link above. For more information, contact Marcia Crosse at (202) 512-7119 or crossem@gao.gov.

In: Safety Efforts in Pediatric Drug Development ISBN: 978-1-60741-565-7
Editor: Conor D. Byrne

Chapter 1

FDA's Authority to Ensure That Drugs Prescribed to Children are Safe and Effective

Susan Thaul
Specialist in Drug Safety and Effectiveness

Summary

In 2007 Congress reauthorized two laws allowing the Food and Drug Administration (FDA) to offer financial and regulatory incentives to test their products for use in children. Through the Food and Drug Administration Amendments Act of 2007 (FDAAA, P.L. 110-85), Congress extended both the Best Pharmaceuticals for Children Act (BPCA) and the Pediatric Research Equity Act (PREA) for five years.

About 75% of drugs have not had pediatric studies. The laws address concerns that clinicians must often prescribe drugs for children that FDA has approved only for adult use. Clinicians often take that step believing that the safety and effectiveness demonstrated with adults would hold for younger patients. But studies show that drugs vary in bioavailability in children, which depends on the maturation and development of organs and other factors. Therefore, this off-label prescribing results in some children's receiving ineffective drugs or too much or too little of a potentially useful drug. It may also result in side effects unique to children, or children of specific ages, including effects on growth and development.

The market has not been able to overcome the economic, ethical, legal, and mechanical obstacles that make manufacturers reluctant to conduct these tests. The reauthorized BPCA and PREA represent ongoing involvement of Congress and FDA to address this need. FDA had tried unsuccessfully to spur pediatric drug research through administrative action before 1997. With the FDA Modernization Act of 1997 (FDAMA, P.L. 105-115), Congress provided an incentive: in exchange for a manufacturer's completion of pediatric studies according to an FDA written request, FDA would extend its market exclusivity for that product for six months. BPCA (P.L. 107-109) gave this program a five-year reauthorization in 2002. To get pediatric use information on the drugs that manufacturers were not studying, in 1998, FDA published the Pediatric Rule requiring that manufacturers submit pediatric testing data at the time of all new drug applications. In 2002, a federal court declared the rule invalid, holding that FDA lacked the statutory authority to promulgate it. Congress gave FDA that authority with PREA (P.L. 108-155). PREA covers drugs and biological products and includes provisions for deferrals, waivers, and the required pediatric assessment of an approved marketed product.

Some of the issues the 110th Congress considered remain of concern. Why offer a financial incentive to encourage pediatric studies when FDA has the authority to require them? How does the cost of marketing exclusivity—including the higher prices paid by government—compare with the cost of the needed research? What percentage of drug labeling includes adequate pediatric information because of BPCA and PREA? Does the law provide FDA with sufficient authority to act and does FDA choose to so act? These kinds of questions—determining what information clinicians and consumers need, how to then develop and disseminate it; how to balance carrots and sticks; and how to consider cost and benefit—could not only help the 111th Congress evaluate BPCA and PREA, but also inform its consideration of healthcare reform.

INTRODUCTION

The Food and Drug Administration (FDA) has approved for adult use many drugs never tested in children. Yet clinicians often prescribe them for children believing that the safety and effectiveness demonstrated with adults probably reasonably transfers to younger patients. The data show that this is not always true.

To encourage industry to develop drugs and medical devices for pediatric use, Congress has established three programs. The Food and Drug Administration Amendments Act of 2007 (FDAAA, P.L. 110-85)[1] reauthorized and strengthened two laws addressing drugs—the *Best Pharmaceuticals for Children Act (BPCA) of 2002* and the *Pediatric Research Equity Act (PREA) of 2003*—and enacted a new law addressing devices—the *Pediatric Medical Device Safety and Improvement Act (PMDSIA) of 2007.*

The historical approach of this report allows an understanding of how and why Congress took these steps. Specifically, it:

- describes why research on a drug's pharmacokinetics, safety, and effectiveness in children is necessary;
- presents why the marketplace has not provided sufficient incentive to manufacturers of drugs approved for adult use;
- analyzes how BPCA and PREA evolved from FDA's administrative earlier efforts;
- describes how FDAAA amended BPCA and PREA;
- analyzes the impact BPCA and PREA have had on pediatric drug research; and
- discusses issues, some of which Congress considered leading up to FDAAA, that may form the basis of oversight and evaluative activities.

Other CRS reports address how FDA handles similar issues relating to pediatric use of medical devices.[2]

NEED FOR PEDIATRIC LABELING

A drug cannot be marketed in the United States without Food and Drug Administration (FDA) approval. A manufacturer's application to FDA must include an *Indication for Use* section that describes what the drug does and the clinical condition and population for which it has tested and seeks approval for sale.

To approve a drug, FDA must find that the manufacturer has sufficiently demonstrated the drug's safety and effectiveness for the specific intended indication (rationale for treatment and its context) and population specified in the application.[3] The Federal Food, Drug, and Cosmetic Act (FFDCA) allows a manufacturer to promote or advertise a drug only for uses listed in the FDA-approved labeling—and the labeling may list only those claims for which FDA has reviewed (and accepted) safety and effectiveness evidence.

However, the FFDCA does not give FDA authority to regulate the practice of medicine; that responsibility rests with the states and medical professional associations. Once FDA approves a drug, therefore, a licensed physician may—except in highly regulated circumstances—prescribe it without restriction. When a clinician prescribes it to an individual whose demographic or medical characteristics differ from those indicated in a drug's FDA-approved labeling, that is called off-label use, which is considered accepted medical practice.

Most of the prescriptions that physicians write for children fall into the category of off-label use. FDA has evaluated the drugs' safety and effectiveness when used to treat adults, but has not seen data relating to their use in children—and thus the labeling does not address indications, dosage, or warnings related to use in children. Faced with an ill child, a clinician must deduce/infer/guess whether the drug might help. The doctor must also decide what dose and how often, all to best balance the drug's intended effect with its anticipated and unanticipated side effects.

Such clinicians face an obstacle: children are not miniature adults.[4] At different ages, a body may handle a given amount of an administered drug differently, resulting in varying bioavailability. This occurs, in part, because the rate at which the body eliminates a drug (after which the drug is no longer available) varies, among other things, on changes in the maturation and development of organs. Clearance can be quicker or slower in children depending on the age of child, the organs involved, and body surface area.[5]

Without complete information on which to make these decisions, clinicians sometimes err. Such errors, as outlined by the Director of FDA's Office of Pediatric Therapeutics, include unnecessary exposure to ineffective drugs; ineffective dosing of an effective drug; overdosing of an effective drug; undefined unique pediatric adverse events; and effects on growth and behavior.[6] **Table 1** includes some of the examples that FDA scientists have included in recent presentations on pediatric drug development.

Such examples demonstrate the need for studies in children of each drug's pharmacokinetics—the uptake, distribution, binding, elimination, and biotransformation rates within the body. Those studies are particularly valuable because doses for some drugs must be *larger* than the adult dose to be effective in children, and because there is great pharmacokinetic variation among children of different ages.

Table 1. Examples of Differences in Effectiveness, Dosing, and Adverse Events for Children Administered Adult-Tested, FDA-Approved Medications

Type of difference	Examples of the need for pediatric labeling
Inability to demonstrate effectiveness	• some cancer drugs • buspirone (Buspar) for general anxiety disorder • some combination diabetes drugs
Children require higher doses than adults	• gabapentin (Neurontin) for seizures: in children less than 5 years old • fluvoxamine (Luvox) for obsessive compulsive disorder (OCD): in adolescents (12 17 year olds) • benazepril (Lotensin) for hypertension
Children require lower doses than adults	• famotidine (Pepcid) for gastroesophageal reflux: in patients less than 3 months of age • fluvoxamine (Luvox) for OCD: in 8-11 year old girls
Unique pediatric adverse events	• betamethasone (Diprolene AF, Lotrisone) for some dermatoses: not recommended in patients less than 12 years of age due to hypopituitary adrenal (HPA) axis suppression
Effects on growth and development	• atomoxetine (Strattera) for attention deficit hyperactivity disorder • fluoxetine (Prozac) for depression and OCD • ribaviron/intron A (Rebetron) for chronic hepatitis C

Sources: Presentations by Drs. Dianne Murphy and William Rodriguez, FDA.

To sum up: Clinicians need pediatric-specific information in the FDA-approved labeling of drugs to help them decide which, if any, drug to use, in what amount, and by what route to administer the drug. They—and their patients' parents or guardians—need to know what range of adverse events have been noted. That information would come from well-designed and well-conducted studies in children—studies that have been slow to appear.

Manufacturers Have Been Reluctant to Test Drugs in Children

Depending on how one defines the denominator (e.g., all drugs, or all drugs used by children), an estimated 65-80% of drugs have not been tested in children. Why not? The market has not been able to overcome the obstacles—which could be economic, ethical, legal, or mechanical—that make manufacturers reluctant to conduct these tests.

The market for any individual drug's pediatric indications is generally small, providing an economic disincentive for manufacturers to commit resources to pediatric testing. Because young children cannot swallow tablets, the manufacturer might have a mechanical hurdle in developing different formulation (such as a liquid). The ethical and legal difficulties encountered in recruiting adult participants in clinical trials are even greater when seeking children: many parents do not want their children in experiments. Also, liability concerns include not only injury but difficult-to-calculate lifetime compensation.

Congress has offered incentives to manufacturers for pediatric research for two main reasons. First, it is clear that, in treating sick children, doctors will continue prescribing drugs despite insufficient pediatric-use studies. Second, Congress has generally believed that, despite the difficulty in conducting such studies, children could be better served once the research was done.

The Current Laws Evolved from Earlier Attempts

Before BPCA 2002 and PREA 2003, FDA attempted to spur pediatric drug research through administrative action (see **Table 2**).

1979: Rule on Drug Labeling

In a 1979 rule on drug labeling, FDA established a "Pediatric use" subsection. The rule required that labeling include pediatric dosage information for a drug with a specific pediatric indication [approved use of the drug]. It also required that statements regarding pediatric use for indications approved for adults be based on "substantial evidence derived from adequate and well-controlled studies" or that the labeling include the statement "Safety and effectiveness in children have not been established."[7]

Despite the 1979 rule, most prescription drug labels continued to lack adequate pediatric use information. The requirement for adequate and well-controlled studies deterred many manufacturers who, apparently, did not understand that the rule included a waiver option. FDA, therefore, issued another rule in 1994.

1994: Revised Rule

The revised rule attempted to make clear that the "adequate and well-controlled studies" language did not require that manufacturers conduct clinical trials in children. The new rule described how FDA would determine whether the evidence was substantial and adequate. If, for example, clinicians would use the drug to treat a different condition in children than its FDA-approved use in adults, FDA would require trials in children. However, if the drug would be used in children for the same condition for which FDA had approved its use in adults, the labeling statement regarding effectiveness could be based on adult trials alone. In such instances, FDA might also require pediatric study-based data on pharmacokinetics or relevant safety measures. The 1994 rule continued the 1979 requirement that manufacturers include statements regarding uses for which there was no substantial evidence of safety and effectiveness. It added a requirement that labels include information about known specific hazards from the active or inactive ingredients.[8]

Table 2. Administrative and Statutory Efforts to Encourage Pediatric Drug Research

Year	Action
1977	FDA pediatric guidance on "General Considerations for the Clinical Evaluation of Drugs in Infants and Children"
1979	FDA rule on *Pediatric Use* subsection of product package insert: Precautions section [21 CFR 201.57(f)(9)] (in 44 Fed. Reg. 37434)
1994	FDA rule revised
1996	FDA guidance on "Content and Format of Pediatric Use Section"
1997	Food and Drug Administration Modernization Act (FDAMA, P.L. 105-115), included the Better Pharmaceuticals for Children Act
1998	FDA Pediatric Rule finalized (effective 1999; invalidated 2002)
2001	Adaptation of HHS Subpart D (pediatric) regulations [45 CFR 36 Subpart D] to FDA-regulated research [21 CFR 50 Subpart D]

Table 2. (Continued)

Year	Action
2002	Best Pharmaceuticals for Children Act (BPCA, P.L. 107-109)
2003	Pediatric Research Equity Act (PREA, P.L. 108-155)
2007	FDA Amendments Act of 2007 (FDAAA, P.L. 110-85) reauthorized BPCA and PREA and enacted the Pediatric Medical Device Safety and Improvement Act

Source: Adapted from Steven Hirschfeld, Division of Oncology Drug Products & Division of Pediatric Drug Development, Center for Drug Evaluation and Research (CDER), FDA, "History of Pediatric Labeling," presentation to the Pediatric Oncology Subcommittee of the Oncologic Drugs Advisory Committee, March 4, 2003, athttp://www.fda.gov/?ohrms/?dockets/?ac/?03/?slides/?3927S1_ 01_Hirshfeld%20.ppt.

Food and Drug Administration Modernization Act of 1997

Three years later, Congress took further action. FDAMA (P.L. 105-115), incorporating the provisions introduced as the Better Pharmaceuticals for Children Act, created a Section 505A (21 U.S.C. 355a) in the FFDCA: Pediatric studies of drugs. It provided drug manufacturers an incentive to conduct pediatric use studies on their patented products. If a manufacturer completed a pediatric study according to FDA's written request, which included design, size, and other specifications, FDA would extend its market exclusivity for that product for six months.[9] The law required that the Secretary publish an annual list of FDA-approved drugs for which additional pediatric information might produce health benefits. FDAMA also required that the Secretary prepare a report examining whether the new law enhanced pediatric use information, whether the incentive was adequate, and what the program's economic impact was on taxpayers and consumers.

1997: The Pediatric Rule

Also in 1997, FDA issued a proposed regulation that came to be called the Pediatric Rule.[10] The Pediatric Rule mandated that manufacturers submit pediatric testing data at the time of all new drug applications to FDA. [Note: This concept is the basis of the Pediatric Research Equity Act, discussed in the next section of this report.] The rule went into effect in 1999, prompting a lawsuit again FDA by the Competitive Enterprise Institute and the Association of American Physicians and Surgeons. The plaintiffs claimed that the agency was acting outside its authority in considering off-label uses of approved drugs. In October 2002, a federal court declared the Pediatric Rule invalid, noting that its finding related not to the Rule's policy value but to FDA's statutory authority in promulgating it:

> The Pediatric Rule may well be a better policy tool than the one enacted by Congress (which encourages testing for pediatric use, but does not require it) ... It might reflect the most thoughtful, reasoned, balanced solution to a vexing public health problem. The issue here is not the Rule's wisdom ... The issue is the Rule's statutory authority, and it is this that the court finds wanting.[11]

BPCA 2002 and PREA 2003: Laws to Encourage Pediatric Drug Research

Although other laws (such as those affecting drug development, safety and effectiveness efforts, and general health care and consumer protection) serve to promote or protect the health of children, the Best Pharmaceuticals for Children Act and the Pediatric Research Equity Act authorize the programs most focused on pediatric drug research. To maintain the historical organization of this report, descriptions of the laws as initially enacted in 2002 and 2003 appear in this section. The following section describes the changes that FDAAA 2007 made.

The Best Pharmaceuticals for Children Act of 2002

Pediatric Exclusivity

The Best Pharmaceuticals for Children Act (BPCA, P.L. 107-109), in 2002, reauthorized FDAMA's pediatric exclusivity provisions in FFDCA Section 505A (21 U.S.C. 355a). BPCA 2002 renewed the agency's authority to give an additional six-month period of marketing exclusivity to a manufacturer in return for FDA-requested pediatric use studies and reports. The provisions applied to both new drugs and drugs already on the market.

FDA-NIH Collaboration

Pediatric exclusivity, however, is not relevant to products that are no longer covered by patent or other marketing exclusivity agreements. Also, a patent-holding manufacturer may decline to conduct the FDA-requested study and, therefore, the exclusivity. BPCA 2002, therefore, added provisions to encourage pediatric research in those products.

Off-patent products

BPCA 2002 addressed the first group, which it described as "off-patent," by adding to the Public Health Service Act (PHSA) a new Section 409I (42 U.S.C. 284m). It established an off-patent research fund at NIH for these studies and authorized appropriations of $200 million for FY2002 and such sums as are necessary for each of the five years until the provisions are set to sunset on October 1, 2007.

Sponsor-declined studies

For on-patent drugs whose manufacturers declined FDA's written requests for studies, BPCA 2002 amended the FFDCA Section 505A to allow their referral by FDA to the Foundation for the National Institutes of Health (FNIH) for pediatric studies, creating a second program of FDANIH collaboration.

Other Provisions

- gave priority status to pediatric supplemental applications;
- established an FDA Office of Pediatric Therapeutics;
- defined pediatric age groups to include neonates;
- directed the HHS Secretary to contract with the Institute of Medicine for a review of regulations, federally prepared or supported reports, and federally supported evidence-based research, all relating to research involving children.[12] The IOM report to Congress was to include recommendations on best practices relating to research involving children.

Pediatric Research Equity Act of 2003

Next, Congress turned its attention to the federal court ruling that FDA had overstepped its statutory authority in promulgating the Pediatric Rule. It gave FDA that authority. The Pediatric Research Equity Act of 2003 (PREA, P.L. 108-155) essentially codified the Pediatric Rule by adding to the FFDCA a new Section 505B (21 U.S.C. 355c): Research into pediatric uses for drugs and biological products. Unlike BPCA, which applied only to drugs, PREA applied both to drugs regulated under the FFDCA and to biological products (e.g., vaccines) regulated under the PHSA.

New Applications.

With PREA, a manufacturer had to submit a pediatric assessment whenever it submitted an application to market a new active ingredient, new indication, new dosage form, new dosing regimen, or new route of administration. Congress mandated that the submission be adequate to assess the safety and effectiveness of the product for the claimed indications in all relevant pediatric subpopulations; and that it support dosing and administration for each pediatric subpopulation for which the product is safe and effective. If the disease course and drug effects were sufficiently similar for adults and children, the HHS Secretary could allow extrapolation from adult study data as evidence of pediatric effectiveness, usually supplemented with other data from children, such as pharmacokinetic studies.

The law specified situations in which the Secretary might defer or waive the pediatric assessment requirement, such as when the Secretary believes doctors already know that a drug should never be used by children. In those cases, it directed that the product's labeling include any waiver based on evidence that pediatric use would be unsafe or ineffective.

Products on the Market

When not having pediatric use information on the label could pose significant risks, the Secretary could now require the manufacturer[13] of an approved drug or licensed biologic to submit a pediatric assessment. Such situations could arise when the Secretary found that a marketed product was used by pediatric patients for indications labeled for adults, or that the product might provide children a meaningful therapeutic benefit over the available alternatives. Before requiring the assessment, the Secretary had to issue a written request under FFDCA Section 505A (BPCA, pediatric exclusivity) or PHSA Section 409I (NIH funding mechanisms). Further, the manufacturer must not have agreed to conduct the assessment, and the Secretary had to have stated that the NIH funding programs either did or did not have enough funds to conduct that study.

If the manufacturer did not comply with the Secretary's request, the Secretary could consider the product misbranded. Because Congress wanted to protect adult access to a product under these circumstances, the law set limits on FDA's enforcement options, precluding, for example, the withdrawal of approval or license to market.

Other Provisions

Seeing PREA and BPCA as complementary approaches to the same goal, Congress, in 2003, linked PREA to BPCA. [Note: A discussion of this linkage appears later in this report.] Therefore, rather than specify a sunset date, Congress authorized PREA to continue only as long as BPCA was in effect.

Comparison of BPCA and PREA

When presenting material about the pediatric research provisions in law, more than one FDA speaker has referred to "the carrot and the stick." BPCA offers a carrot—extended market exclusivity in return for specific studies on pediatric use; PREA follows up with a stick—required studies of a drug's safety and effectiveness when used by children. **Table 3**, adapted from an FDA slide presentation, summarizes the key differences between these two laws.

Table 3. Major Differences in the BPCA and PREA Approaches

BPCA	PREA
Added FFDCA Section 505A	Added FFDCA Section 505B
Pediatric research	Pediatric assessments
Pediatric studies are voluntary and in exchange for marketing exclusivity	Pediatric studies are mandatory
Applies to drugs	Applies to drugs and biologics
Research and exclusivity to cover all uses of the active drug component	Research to cover the indicated use, dose, and route of administration under FDA review

Source: Adapted from Lisa Mathis, Associate Director, Pediatric and Maternal Health Team, Office of New Drugs, CDER, "Growth and Development of Pediatric Drug Development at the FDA," June 2006 presentation to the Institute of Medicine, the National Academies, at http://www.fda.gov/?oc/?opt/?presentations/?drugdevelopment.ppt.

PEDIATRIC PROVISIONS IN FDAAA 2007

Five years after passing BPCA and PREA, in a year that saw rising concern about drug safety, Congress reauthorized BPCA and thereby also continued PREA. Much of the two laws remained the same, and Congress added provisions to strengthen the programs. What follows groups the changes placed in the FDA Amendments Act of 2007.[14]

Best Pharmaceuticals for Children Act of 2007

Pediatric Exclusivity

BPCA 2007 (Title V of FDAAA) again reauthorized the pediatric exclusivity program, amending FFDCA 505A to sunset on October 1, 2012. Its provisions encourage research on off-patent products, strengthen the requirements for labeling changes based on the results of pediatric use studies, and provide for the reporting of adverse events.

Internal Review Committee

- required that the Secretary establish an internal review committee, composed of FDA employees with specified expertise, to review all written requests; and
- required the Secretary, with that committee, to track pediatric studies and labeling changes according to specified questions.

Study Requirements

- refined study scope to allow the Secretary to include preclinical studies; and
- required supporting evidence if an applicant turned down a request on the grounds that developing appropriate pediatric formulations of the drug was not possible.

Reporting, Labeling, and Timing

- authorized the Secretary to grant additional marketing exclusivity, for both new drugs and drugs already on the market, only after: a sponsor completed and reported on the studies that the Secretary had requested in writing; the studies included appropriate formulations of the drug for each age group of interest; and any appropriate labeling changes were approved; all within the agreed upon time frames; and
- required that the sponsor propose pediatric labeling resulting from the studies.

Adverse Event Reports

- required applicants to submit, along with the report of requested studies, all postmarket adverse event reports regarding that drug.

Required Public Notice

- expanded the public notice requirement beyond the current notice of an exclusivity decision to include copies of the written request;
- required the Secretary to publicly identify any drug with a developed pediatric formulation that studies had shown were safe and effective for children that an applicant has not brought to market within one year;
- required that, for a product studied under this section, the labeling include study results (if they do or do not indicate safety and effectiveness, or if they are inconclusive) and the Secretary's determination;
- required dissemination of labeling change information to health-care providers; and
- required reporting on the review of all adverse event reports and recommendations to the Secretary on actions in response.

Dispute Resolution

- established a dispute resolution process to include referral to the Pediatric Advisory Committee.

FDA-NIH Collaboration

Off-Patent Products

- required the Secretary to determine (in consultation with an internal committee required by FDAAA) whether there is a continuing need for pediatric studies. If so, the Secretary must refer those drugs for inclusion on the list of priority needs in pediatric therapeutics that require study;
- amended PHSA Section 409I (as discussed earlier), which required that the Secretary, through the NIH Director and in consultation with the FDA Commissioner and pediatric research experts, list approved drugs for which pediatric studies are needed to assess safety and effectiveness. It changed the specifications from an annual list of approved drugs to a list,

revised every three years, of priority study needs in pediatric therapeutics, including drugs or indications;

- for drugs for which pediatric studies are not completed and for which the Secretary determines there is a need for pediatric information, required the Secretary to determine whether funds are available through the Foundation for the NIH. If yes, required Secretary to issue a proposal to award a grant to conduct such studies. If no, required the Secretary to refer the drug for inclusion on the list established under PHSA Section 409I;
- required reports from the Institute of Medicine and the Government Accountability Office; and
- included the same authorization of appropriations.

Sponsor-Declined Studies

- required the Secretary, after determining that an on-patent drug requires pediatric study, to determine whether the FNIH has sufficient money to fund a grant or contract for such studies. If it does, the Secretary must refer that study to FNIH and FNIH must fund it. If FNIH has insufficient funds, the Secretary may require the manufacturer to conduct a pediatric assessment under PREA. If the Secretary does not require the study, the Secretary must notify the public of that decision and the reasons for it.

Other Provisions

- made ineligible for exclusivity any drug with another exclusivity due to expire in less than nine months.

Pediatric Research Equity Act of 2007

Next, in order to preserve the carrot and stick approach to encouraging pediatric research, Congress not only reauthorized the Pediatric Research Equity Act (PREA 2007, Title IV of FDAAA) but also amended it to strengthen standards for required tests, explanation of deferrals, labeling, and publicly accessible information.

New Applications

PREA 2007 required manufacturers to provide documentation of the data used to support extrapolation of effectiveness findings from adult studies to pediatric age groups.

Products on the Market

PREA 2007 continued the Secretary's authority to require a manufacturer to submit require assessments. It described the circumstances somewhat differently. PREA 2002 applied to a drug used to treat a substantial number of pediatric patients for the labeled indications, and for which the *absence* of adequate labeling could pose *significant risks* to pediatric patients. PREA 2007, however:

- applied to a drug used for a substantial number of pediatric patients for the labeled indications, and for which the *presence* of adequate pediatric labeling "could confer a *benefit* on pediatric patients;" and
- covered a situation in which there was reason to believe the drug would represent a meaningful therapeutic benefit over existing therapies for pediatric patients for one or more of the claimed indications.

Adding to the procedure for when the Secretary grants a *deferral* of some of all of the requirement assessments, PREA 2007:

- required that the applicant include a timeline for the completion of such studies;
- required the Secretary's annual review of each approved deferral, for which the applicant must submit evidence of documentation of study progress; and
- required that all information from that review promptly be made available to the public.

Regarding *waiver* of the requirement to develop a pediatric formulation, PREA 2007:

- required the manufacturer to submit documentation detailing why a pediatric formulation could not be developed; and
- required that submitted materials for granted waivers promptly be made available to the public.

Other Provisions

PREA 2007:

- required that the Secretary establish an internal committee, composed of FDA employees with specified expertise, to participate in the review of pediatric plans and assessments, deferrals, and waivers;
- required the Secretary to track assessments and labeling changes and to make that information publicly accessible;
- established a dispute resolution procedure, which would allow the Commissioner, after specified steps, to deem a drug to be misbranded if a manufacturer refused to make a requested labeling change;
- included review and reporting requirements for adverse events;
- required reports from both the Institute of Medicine (IOM) and the Government Accountability Office (GAO); and
- continued to link the program's authorization to the five-year authority FDAAA provides to the pediatric exclusivity program.

BPCA AND PREA IMPACT ON PEDIATRIC DRUG RESEARCH

FDA maintains statistics on the two pediatric research encouragement programs on the FDA website.[15]

Best Pharmaceuticals for Children Act

On-Patent Drugs

The FDA website offers regularly updated data on activity related to BPCA. **Table 4** uses some of those data.[16] Through October 31, 2008, FDA had issued 360 written requests for pediatric studies to manufacturers holding patent or other exclusivity benefits. The requests, which outlined 854 specific studies, also specified the study purpose: about half of the studies addressed efficacy and safety, and more than a third focused on aspects of pharmacokinetics.

Of those 360 written requests, FDA has made exclusivity determinations for 48% (n = 171), noting that the manufacturer has completed and submitted reports on the requested studies. It granted pediatric exclusivity to 92% (n = 157) of those, representing 151 active components. Through November 5, 2008, FDA attributed 157 labeling changes (involving 150 drugs) to BPCA.[17]

Table 4. Pediatric Exclusivity Statistics

	Number
FDA written requests	360
Exclusivity determinations	171
Drugs granted exclusivity	157
Labeling changed	150

Source: CRS presentation of FDA data, at http://www.fda.gov/?cder/?pediatric.

Of the 360 written requests, 52% (n = 190) have not progressed to an exclusivity determination. For those drugs, studies may be in progress or the manufacturers may have chosen not to accept exclusivity and the pediatric study requirements. Therefore, only 42% of the 360 requests have yielded pediatric labeling changes.

NIH Route for Off-Patent Drugs and On-Patent Drugs for Which Manufacturers Declined FDA's Requests for Study

Under BPCA, the NIH list has 57 drug-indication entries.[18] NIH has recommended that no studies be pursued for 11 (19%) of those. **Table 5** divides the remaining 46 drugs recommended for pediatric study from 2003 through March 2007 by patent status and whether a study had begun. Thirteen (28%) have progressed to choice of clinical trial sites, an indication that they are funded.

GAO Study

In March 2007, the Government Accountability Office (GAO) issued a report that the BPCA legislation had required.[19] Noting that most of the exclusivity-associated studies resulted in labeling changes, GAO calculated the time that elapsed before those changes were completed. The entire process—from initial data submission, through FDA review and frequent requests for additional data, to follow-up submissions and reviews—took an average of nine months. Onethird of the drugs' labeling changing took less than three months, while labeling change for one took almost three years. The GAO report identified three main categories of labeling change: to inform of ineffective drugs, dosing that was too high or too low, and newly identified adverse events. It juxtaposed those findings with the statement that children take many of these drugs for common, serious, or life-threatening conditions.

Pediatric Research Equity Act

FDA has approved more than 500 new drug and biologics license applications since the beginning of 2003.[20] For that same period, FDA attributes 88 labeling changes to PREA.[21] **Table 5** indicates the topics of those label changes.

Table 5. Research Status of Drugs That NIH Deemed In Need of Pediatric Studies, by Patent Status

Clinical trial site chosen			Total[Error! Reference source not found.]
Patent status	**Yes**	**No**	
On	4 (29%)	10	14
Off	9 (28%)	23	32
Total	13 (28%)	33	46

a. Total excludes the 11 off-patent products for which NIH does not recommend further study at this time.

Source: NICHD, "Table 1: Current Status of Drugs Which Have Been Listed by NIH (NICHD) for BPCA As of March 28, 2007," BPCA, athttp://bpca.nichd.nih.gov/?about/?process/?upload/ ?Drug_Table_2007.pdf.

Table 6. Content of PREA-Associated Labeling Changes

Topic of label change	Number of label changes
Extended indication	5
New active ingredient	14
New dosage form	26
New dosing regimen	10
New drug	5
New indication	25
New route of administration	3
Total number of label changes[a]	**88**

a. The 88 changes apply to 76 products; 12 products had two label changes (e.g., Xopenex HFA Inhalation Aerosol had both a new active ingredient and an extended indication).

Source: FDA, "PREA Labeling Changes," updated August 8, 2008, at http://www.fda.gov/?CDER/?pediatric/?PREA_label_post-mar_2_mtg.pdf.

FDA Activities

In its implementation of the pediatric research laws, FDA has published many documents and provides electronic links to these documents on its "Pediatric Drug

Development" page, at http://www.fda.gov/?cder/?pediatric/. These include the following:

- **Rules and announcements,** such as "Summaries of Medical and Clinical Pharmacology Reviews of Pediatric Studies; Availability," *Federal Register*, vol. 73, no. 45, March 6, 2008, pp. 12182-12183.
- **Final and draft guidances,** such as *Qualifying for Pediatric Exclusivity Under Section 505A of the Federal Food, Drug, and Cosmetic Act*, issued in 1999; and *How to Comply with the Pediatric Research Equity Act*, draft issued in 2005.
- **Written request templates,** such as "Sample Written Request For Division of Oncology Drug Products."
- **Agenda and transcripts for the meetings of advisory committees,** such as "FDA Pediatric Ethics Working Group Consensus Statement on the Pediatric Advisory Subcommittee's April 24, 2001 Meeting."
- **Statistics,** such as "Pediatric Exclusivity Labeling Changes as of November 5, 2008," and "PREA Labeling Changes," updated August 8, 2008.

Recurring Issues for Congress

Because Congress has reauthorized BPCA and PREA and passed PMDSIA, it may wait for their 2012 reauthorizations before taking further legislative action in this area. Meanwhile, regardless of legislative possibilities, there remain concerns about exclusivity, cost, labeling, enforcement, and sunsets. This report concludes by reviewing each.

Exclusivity

BPCA offers pharmaceutical companies a reward for agreeing to conduct studies on drugs for pediatric populations. But PREA requires pediatric studies.

Some may ask why Congress must offer industry a reward for something it requires them to do.

After reviewing the history of pediatric exclusivity during the period when Congress was considering reauthorizing the FDAMA exclusivity provisions in a proposed BPCA, one legal analyst wrote, in 2003:

> If Congress had codified the FDA's power to require testing in all new and already marketed drugs, the notion of an incentive or reward for testing would appear ludicrous.[22]

In fact, Congress did exactly that: provided an incentive for something that is already a requirement. During the debate on PREA in 2003, Members of the Senate clearly had questions about this contradiction.[23] While Senator Gregg, as committee chair, wrote: "The Pediatric Rule was intended to work as a safety net to (or as a backstop to) pediatric exclusivity;" Senator Clinton and others wrote in the report's "Additional Views" section:

> Neither the intent conveyed by FDA nor FDA's implementation of the [Pediatric] [R]ule supports the report's contention that the rule was intended to work as a 'backstop' to pediatric exclusivity or to be employed only to fill the gaps in coverage left by the exclusivity.

Three years later, in its draft guidance on "How to Comply with the Pediatric Research Equity Act," FDA wrote that "[t]he Pediatric Rule was designed to work in conjunction with the pediatric exclusivity provisions of section 505A of the Act...." The BPCA and PREA reauthorizations in 2007 did not change their relationship.

The contradiction remained, continued by FDAAA 2007, and is now law. At some point Congress may want to resolve this apparent paradox.

Cost

In assessing the value of BPCA and PREA, it may be useful to identify the intended and unintended effects—both positive and negative—of their implementation. Let us say FDA grants a manufacturer a six-month exclusivity. Who benefits?

The manufacturer. The manufacturer holding pediatric exclusivity incurs the research and development expenses related to the FDA-requested pediatric studies. It then enjoys six months of sales without a competitor product and a potentially lucrative head start on future sales.

Other manufacturers. The manufacturers that do not hold the exclusivity, must wait six months during which they cannot launch competing products. After that, however, they may be able to market generic versions of a drug that has been assessed for pediatric use and has had six months' experience in the public's awareness.

Government. Nonfinancial benefits to government include its progress in protecting children's health. Costs to the government include administrative and regulatory expenses. Because the government also pays for drugs, both directly and indirectly, it must pay the higher price that exclusivity allows for six months. The better pediatric information, however, may yield future financial savings by avoiding ineffective and unsafe uses.

Private insurers. Private payers also face similar financial costs and benefits as public payers, without the regulatory costs of administering the program.

Children and their families. Some children may incur risks as study subjects; they and others might benefit from more appropriate use of drugs, including accurate dosing.

Although assigning quantitative values to those effects is generally beyond the scope of this report, some researchers have examined the *financial* costs and benefits faced by manufacturers that receive pediatric exclusivity. One study appeared in February 2007, written by a team led by Jennifer Li of Duke University's Department of Pediatrics, with co-authors from its Department of Economics and the Duke Clinical Research Institute, as well as from the Office of the Commissioner at FDA.[24] It calculated the net economic benefit (costs minus benefits, after much estimating and adjusting for other factors) to a manufacturer that, in 2002-2004, responded to an FDA request for pediatric studies and received pediatric exclusivity. The median net economic benefit of six-month exclusivity was $134.3 million. The study found a large range, from a net loss to a net benefit of over half a billion dollars.

Although the BPCA reauthorization in 2007 continued the six-month exclusivity, the Senate bill would have limited the period of exclusivity for a drug to three months if its manufacturer/sponsor had more than $1 billion in annual gross U.S. sales for all its products with the same active ingredient. In future years, Congress might reexamine whether such limits may be in the public interest.

Labeling

Pediatric studies can produce valuable information about safety, effectiveness, dosing, or side effects when a child takes a medication. Such information benefits children only when it reaches clinicians and others who care for children (including parents). BPCA 2002, PREA 2003, and their 2007 reauthorizations, therefore, included labeling provisions to make the information available.

As a result, FDA now requires, by law or regulation, pediatric usage labeling in the following circumstances:

- manufacturer has successfully applied (via an original new drug application
  [NDA] or a supplement) for approval to list a pediatric indication;
- manufacturer has received pediatric exclusivity after conducting appropriate
  studies; or
- manufacturer has submitted the safety and effectiveness findings from pediatric
  assessments required under PREA.

In the first case, the labeling includes pediatric use information only if FDA approved the pediatric indication. If FDA turned down or the manufacturer withdrew a request for a pediatric indication, pediatric use information appears nowhere in the product's labeling. In addition, the fact that the manufacturer had made an unsuccessful attempt—and the research findings that blocked approval—would be neither noted in the label nor made public in other ways.

When it comes to exclusivity, the labeling rules are different. If the studies required for exclusivity support pediatric use or specific limits to pediatric use (different dosing or subgroups), that information would go in the labeling. The labeling would also make clear if the studies did not find the drug to be effective in children or if FDA waived the requirement to study because children should not or would not be given the drug.

The rules have created measurable change. Still, not all drugs used by children have labeling that addresses pediatric use. As previously noted, FDA approved more than 500 new drug and biologics license applications from the beginning of 2003 through September 2008.[25] Yet, the PREA statistics on labeling note 88 labeling changes over that period.

The PREA and BPCA reauthorizations in 2007 added the third circumstance of required pediatric labeling. Upon determining that a pediatric assessment or study does or does not demonstrate that the subject drug is safe and effective in pediatric populations or subpopulations, the Secretary must order the label to include information about those results and a statement of the Secretary's determination. That is true even if the study results were inconclusive.

Labeling is useful if its statements are clear, useful, and read. While an improvement over no mention at all, a statement such as "... effectiveness in pediatric patients has not been established" still deprives a clinician of information that is available. The statement does not distinguish among:

- studies in children found the drug to be ineffective;
- studies in children found the drug to be unsafe;
- studies in children were not conclusive regarding safety or effectiveness; or
- no studies had been conducted concerning pediatric use.

If studies suggest that safety, effectiveness, or dosage reactions vary by age, condition to be treated, or patient circumstances, then detailed information could be included in the labeling. BPCA 2007 also strengthened the effect of labeling requirements by mandating the dissemination of certain safety and effectiveness information to health care providers and the public.

Although not included in the pediatric sections, another provision in FDAAA 2007 may yield benefits for pediatric labeling. Regarding television and radio direct-to-consumer (DTC) drug advertisements, the law required that major statements relating to side effects and contraindications be presented in a clear, conspicuous, and neutral manner. It further required that the Secretary establish standards for determining whether a major statement meets those criteria. The fruits of such inquiry could be applied throughout Agency communication.

Finally, BPCA 2003 had required HHS to promulgate a rule within one year of enactment regarding the placement on all drug labels of a toll-free telephone number with which to report adverse events. FDA issued a proposed rule in 2004 but has not yet finalized it. BPCA 2007 required that the 2004 proposed rule take effect on January 1, 2008 unless the Commissioner issued the final rule before then. It limited the rule's application to exclude certain drugs whose packaging already includes a toll-free number for consumers to report complaints to their manufacturers or distributors.[26]

Enforcement

FDA's postmarket authority regarding pediatric drug use labeling has been limited. Congress had given FDA the authority to use its sledgehammer—deeming a product to be "misbranded" and thereby gaining the authority to pull it from the market—but has not given the agency authority to require less drastic actions, such as labeling changes.

To pull from the market a drug on which many consumers rely would be, according to some health-care analysts, akin to throwing out the baby with the bathwater. In its report accompanying its PREA 2003 bill, the Senate committee noted its intent that the misbranding authority regarding pediatric use labeling not be the basis for criminal proceedings or withdrawal of approval, and only rarely result in seizure of the offending product.[27] The 2007 reauthorization continues this approach.

Again outside its pediatric-specific sections, FDAAA created a new enforcement authority for FDA: civil monetary penalties. Framed in the context of giving FDA tools to create meaningful incentives for manufacturer compliance with a range of postmarket safety activities, the provision listed labeling within its scope. In Senate and House committee discussions of what maximum penalties to allow, proposed one-time penalties were as low as $15,000 and proposed upper levels ranged to $50 million. The final provision says that an applicant violating certain requirements regarding postmarket safety, studies or clinical trials, *or labeling* is subject to a civil monetary penalty of not more than $250,000 per violation, and not to exceed $1 million for all such violations adjudicated in a single proceeding. If a violation continues after the Secretary provides notice of such violation to the applicant, the Secretary may impose a civil penalty of $250,000 for the first 30 days, doubling for every subsequent 30-day period, up to $1 million for one 30-day period, and up to $10 million for all such violations adjudicated in a single proceeding. The Secretary must, in determining the amount of civil penalty, consider whether the sponsor is making efforts toward correcting the violation.

What options should FDA have if a manufacturer that has already received the six-month pediatric exclusivity then refuses or delays making an appropriate labeling change? For studies that result in labeling changes, when should FDA make study results available to the public?

In considering whether to strengthen FDA's enforcement authority within the context of pediatric research and labeling, Congress can address manufacturers' actions at many points in the regulatory process, if and when, for example, FDA notes: a manufacturer's reluctance to accept the agency's requested study scope, design, and timetable; that a study's completion is clearly lagging or overdue; that a manufacturer does not complete such a study; or does not release its results to FDA, peer-reviewed publications, or the public; or that procedures to incorporate pediatric study results into a drug's labeling have not proceeded appropriately.

There are actions, as well, for the Secretary. BCPA 2007 expanded the Secretary's authority and, in some cases, requires action. The Secretary must publish within 30 days of the Secretary's determination regarding market exclusivity and must include a copy of the written request that specified what studies were necessary. The Secretary must also publicly identify any drug with a developed pediatric formulation that studies have demonstrated to be safe and effective for children if its sponsor has not introduced the pediatric formulation onto the market within one year.

Sunset

Not every law contains a sunset provision. BPCA does, and, although it doesn't use the term, Congress structured PREA 2003 to cease if and when BPCA did. By including an end date or another indication of a predetermined termination date, Congress provides "an 'action-forcing' mechanism, carrying the ultimate threat of termination, and a framework or guidelines for the systematic review and evaluation of past performance."[28]

The sunset provision for BPCA's exclusivity incentive to manufacturers has not engendered congressional debate. During PREA consideration in 2003, however, some Members had objected, unsuccessfully, to linking PREA's safety and effectiveness assessment and resulting pediatric labeling to the BPCA sunset. By the committee markups of PREA in 2007, some Members advocated making the mandatory pediatric assessments permanent. If Congress intended the PREA sunset to trigger regular evaluation of the law's usefulness, there may be other legislative approaches that would more directly achieve that.

If, however, the intent was to test the idea of requiring pediatric assessments, the past five years had provided satisfactory evidence.[29] The House-passed bill would have eliminated PREA's link to the BPCA sunset provision; the Senate-passed bill continued it. The enacted bill included the linkage written in the 2003 legislation. At some point, Congress may wish to evaluate the usefulness and effect of that link.

Concluding Comments

Congress has now repeatedly acted to encourage research into the unique effects of FDA-regulated drugs on children—with both carrots of financial incentive and sticks of required action. It has also required that drug labeling reflect the findings of pediatric research, whether positive, negative, or inconclusive. And, most recently, it has given FDA broader authority to follow up and enforce these requirements.

With each step of legislative and regulatory action over the years, Congress and FDA have tried to balance goals that often conflict:

- drug development to address needs unique to children;
- tools to encourage drug manufacturers to do this, despite the expense, opportunity costs, and liability risk;
- public access to up-to-date and unbiased information on drug safety and effectiveness;
- pharmaceutical industry needs; and
- adequate funding.

Concerns remain, though, about many of the issues discussed during last year's reauthorizations—and in the last section of this paper. Against the backdrop of this fall's financial crisis and the uncertainty about how that will affect the priorities of a new President and Congress, it is hard to predict whether the 111th Congress will wish to address them. They may surface only when reauthorizations are due in 2012.

But the likely legislative debate over health care reform offers Congress opportunities to further ensure safe and effective drugs for children. Some proposed reform elements, such as transparency and evidence-based decisions, already appear in BPCA and PREA. For pediatric drugs, using the appropriate dose for the appropriate illness for the appropriate patient is not only good health care but avoids expensive unnecessary, ineffective, or unsafe treatment. Assessing the administrative and research success (or drawbacks) of the BPCA and PREA programs could inform congressional debate over health care organization and financing to help control the cost of reforms that attempt to broaden access to care.

Author Contact Information

Susan Thaul
Specialist in Drug Safety and Effectiveness
sthaul@crs.loc.gov, 7-0562

End Notes

[1]CRS Report RL34465, *FDA Amendments Act of 2007 (P.L. 110-85)*, by Erin D. Williams and Susan Thaul, presents detailed descriptions of these and other FDAAA provisions.

[2] CRS Report RL32826, *The Medical Device Approval Process and Related Legislative Issues*, and CRS Report RL33981, *Medical Device User Fee and Modernization Act (MDUFMA) Reauthorization*, both by Erin D. Williams.

[3] For descriptions and discussions of the FDA procedure for approving new drugs, seeCRS Report RL32797, *Drug Safety and Effectiveness: Issues and Action Options After FDA Approval*, by Susan Thaul, and FDA, "Drug Approval Application Process," at http://www.fda.gov /?cder/?regulatory/?applications/?default.htm.

[4] David A. Williams, Haiming Xu, and Jose A. Cancelas, "Children are not little adults: just ask their hematopoietic stem cells," *J Clin Invest.*, vol. 116, no. 10, October 2, 2006, pp. 2593-2596; and Stephen Ashwal (Editor), *The Founders of Child Neurology* (San Francisco: Norman Publishing, 1990).

[5] William Rodriguez, Office of New Drugs, FDA, "What We Learned from the Study of Drugs Under the Pediatric Initiatives," June 2006 presentation to the Institute of Medicine, at http://www.fda.gov/?oc/?opt/?presentations/?whatwelearned.ppt.

[6] Dianne Murphy, Director, Office of Pediatric Therapeutics, Office of the Commissioner, FDA, "Impact of Pediatric Legislative Initiatives: USA," January 26, 2005 presentation to the European Forum for Good Clinical Practice, at http://www.fda.gov/?oc/?opt/ ?presentations/?Brussels.ppt; and Rodriguez, June 2006.

[7] FDA, "Labeling and Prescription Drug Advertising; Content and Format for Labeling for Human Prescription Drugs; Final rule," *Federal Register*, vol. 44, no. 124, June 26, 1979, pp. 37434-37467.

[8] FDA, "Specific Requirements on Content and Format of Labeling for Human Prescription Drugs; Revision of "Pediatric Use" Subsection In the Labeling; Final rule," *Federal Register*, vol. 59, no. 238, December 13, 1994, pp. 64240-64250.

[9] Although market exclusivity is a characteristic of patent benefit, the FDA-granted exclusivity is not a patent extension; rather, it means that, during the six-month period, FDA would not grant marketing approval to another identical product (usually a generic). For more discussion of pharmaceutical patents and marketing exclusivity, see, for example, CRS Report RL33288, *Proprietary Rights in Pharmaceutical Innovation: Issues at the Intersection of Patents and Marketing Exclusivities*, by John R. Thomas.

[10] FDA, "Regulations Requiring Manufacturers to Assess the Safety and Effectiveness of New Drugs and Biological Products in Pediatric Patients; Final rule," *Federal Register*, vol. 63, no. 231, December 2, 1998, pp. 66632-66672.

[11] U.S. District Judge Henry H. Kennedy Jr. quoted in Marc Kaufman, "Judge Rejects Drug Testing on Children; Ruling Finds FDA Overstepped Authority in Forcing Pediatric Studies," *Washington Post*, October 19, 2002, p. A9.

[12] See Institute of Medicine, *Ethical Conduct of Clinical Research Involving Children*, Committee on Clinical Research Involving Children (Washington, DC: National Academies Press, 2004), done with funding from NIH and FDA.

[13] The laws refer to the *sponsor* of an application or the *holder* of an approved application. Because that entity is usually the product's manufacturer, this report uses the term *manufacturer* throughout.

[14] CRS Report RL34465, *FDA Amendments Act of 2007 (P.L. 110-85)*, by Erin D. Williams and Susan Thaul, presents detailed tables comparing FDAAA 2007 with BPCA 2002 and PREA 2003, showing both changed and unchanged provisions.

[15] FDA, "Pediatric Drug Development," at http://www.fda.gov/?cder/?pediatric.

[16] FDA, "Drugs to Which FDA has Granted Pediatric Exclusivity for Pediatric Studies under Section 505A of the Federal Food, Drug, and Cosmetic Act," updated November 13, 2008, at http://www.fda.gov/?cder/?pediatric/?exgrant.htm; "Pediatric Exclusivity Labeling Changes as of November 5, 2008," at http://www.fda.gov/?cder/?pediatric/?labelchange.htm; "Pediatric Exclusivity Statistics as of October 31, 2008," at http://www.fda.gov/?cder/?pediatric /?wrstats.htm; and "Studies Breakdown Report for Issued Written Requests as of October 31, 2008: Pediatric Exclusivity," at http://www.fda.gov/?cder /?pediatric/?breakdown.htm.

[17] Staff in the FDA Office of Legislation (telephone communication, November 25, 2008) noted the coincidence of 157 products with exclusivity and the 157 labeling changes. Studies can yield information for labeling changes although FDA did not grant the product exclusivity.

[18] National Institute of Child Health and Human Development, "Best Pharmaceuticals for Children Act: Status of Drugs Listed by NICHD," at http://bpca.nichd.nih.gov/?about/?Process /?status.cfm.

[19] Government Accountability Office (GAO), *Pediatric Drug Research: Studies Conducted under Best Pharmaceuticals for Children Act,* Report to Congressional Committees, GAO-07-557, March 2007.

[20] FDA, "CDER Approval Times for Priority and Standard NDAs and BLAs, Calendar Years 1993-2006," January 29, 2007, at http://www.fda.gov/?cder/?rdmt/?NDAapps93-06.htm; "CDER Drug and Biologic Approvals for Calendar Year 2007," at http://www.fda.gov/?cder/?rdmt/?InternetNDA07.htm, and "CDER Drug and Biologic Approvals for Calendar Year 2008, Updated through September 30, 2008," at http://www.fda.gov/?cder/?rdmt/?InternetNDA08.htm. FDA's Center for Drug Evaluation and Research has, since 2004, covered Biologics License Applications (BLAs) for therapeutic biologics [e.g., monoclonal antibodies for in vivo use; most proteins intended for therapeutic use, including cytokines (e.g., interferons), enzymes (e.g. thrombolytics), and other novel proteins; immunomodulators; and growth factors]; other BLAs [e.g., vaccines, blood products, and coagulation factors], which are regulated within FDA's Center for Biologics Evaluation and Research, are not included in this tally.

[21] FDA, "PREA Labeling Changes," updated August 8, 2008, at http://www.fda.gov/?CDER/?pediatric/?PREA_label_post-mar_2_mtg.pdf.

[22] Lauren Hammer Breslow, "The Best Pharmaceuticals for Children Act of 2002: The Rise of the Voluntary Incentive Structure and Congressional Refusal to Require Pediatric Testing," *Harvard Journal on Legislation*, vol. 40, 2003, pp. 133-191.

[23] S.Rept. 108-84, to accompany S. 650, the Pediatric Research Equity Act of 2003, June 27, 2003.

[24] Jennifer S. Li, Eric L. Eisenstein, Henry G. Grabowski, et al., "Economic Return of Clinical Trials Performed Under the Pediatric Exclusivity Program," *Journal of the American Medical Association*, vol. 297, no. 5, February 7, 2007, pp. 480-488.

[25] For more information, see http://www.fda.gov/?cder/?rdmt/?NDAapps93-06.htm.

[26] FDA issued the final rule on October 28, 2008. Its effective date is November 28, 2008, and its compliance date is July 1, 2009 (FDA [21 CFR Parts 201, 208, and 209], "Toll-Free Number for Reporting Adverse Events on Labeling for Human Drug Products; Final rule," *Federal Register*, v. 73, no. 209, October 28, 2008, pp. 63886-63897).

[27] S.Rept. 108-84.

[28] CRS Report RS21210, *Sunset Review: A Brief Introduction*, by Virginia A. McMurtry.

[29] See Senator Clinton's comments at the Senate Committee on Health, Education, Labor, and Pensions hearing, "Ensuring Safe Medicines and Medical Devices for Children," March 27, 2007,athttp://www.cq.com/?display.do?dockey=/?cqonline/?prod/?data/?docs/?html/?transcripts /?congressional/?110/?congres sionaltranscripts110- 000002481833.html@ committees &metapub =CQCONGTRANSCRIPTS&searchIndex=0&seqNum=13; and S.Rept. 108-84, AdditionalViews.

In: Safety Efforts in Pediatric Drug Development ISBN: 978-1-60741-565-7
Editor: Conor D. Byrne

Chapter 2

GUIDANCE FOR INDUSTRY[1] NONCLINICAL SAFETY EVALUATION OF PEDIATRIC DRUG PRODUCTS

U.S. Dept. of Health and Human Services, Food and Drug Administration, Centre for Drug Evaluation and Research (CDER)

This guidance represents the Food and Drug Administration's (FDA's) current thinking on this topic. It does not create or confer any rights for or on any person and does not operate to bind FDA or the public. You can use an alternative approach if the approach satisfies the requirements of the applicable statutes and regulations. If you want to discuss an alternative approach, contact the FDA staff responsible for implementing this guidance. If you cannot identify the appropriate FDA staff, call the appropriate number listed on the title page of this guidance.

I. INTRODUCTION

This document provides guidance on the role and timing of animal studies in the nonclinical safety evaluation of therapeutics intended for the treatment of pediatric patients. The guidance discusses some conditions under which juvenile animals can be meaningful predictors of toxicity in pediatric patients and makes recommendations on nonclinical testing.

The scope of this guidance is limited to safety effects that cannot be adequately, ethically, and safely assessed in pediatric clinical trials. Serious adverse effects that are irreversible are of particular concern. The guidance also makes recommendations on the timing and utility of juvenile animal studies in relation to phases of clinical development. Sponsors are encouraged to communicate with the appropriate review division to determine whether a juvenile animal study is needed for a particular drug product and to discuss protocol designs before study initiation.

FDA's guidance documents, including this guidance, do not establish legally enforceable responsibilities. Instead, guidances describe the Agency's current thinking on a topic and should be viewed only as recommendations, unless specific regulatory or statutory requirements are cited. The use of the word *should* in Agency guidances means that something is suggested or recommended, but not required.

II. Background

Many therapeutics marketed in the United States and used in pediatric patients lack adequate information in the labeling for use in that population. A survey conducted by the American Academy of Pediatrics shows that the majority of the drugs listed in the *Physician's Desk Reference* lack information on safety and/or efficacy for pediatric use (Committee on Drugs, American Academy of Pediatrics 1995). However, recent pediatric legislation, including the Best Pharmaceuticals for Children Act (BPCA 2002) and the Pediatric Research Equity Act (PREA 2003), have provided a mechanism to obtain the needed pediatric safety and efficacy information in drug product labels.

Drug development programs have used safety data from clinical studies in adults, supported by nonclinical studies in adult animals, to support the use of a drug in pediatric patients. This assumes that pediatric patients will exhibit similar disease progression, and respond similarly to the intended therapeutic intervention. It is clear, however, that these studies may not always assess possible drug effects on developmental processes specific to pediatric age groups. Developmental processes in pediatric patients may differentially affect drug pharmacokinetics and pharmacodynamics compared to adult therapeutic use. Some adverse effects may be very difficult to detect in clinical trials or during routine postmarketing surveillance. Data obtained from clinical pediatric initiatives have identified ineffective dosing and overdosing of effective drugs as well as unnecessary exposure to ineffective therapies and identification of novel pediatric adverse events. Juvenile animal studies may assist in identifying postnatal developmental toxicities that are not adequately assessed in reproductive toxicity assessments and that may not be adequately and safely tested in pediatric clinical trials.

III. General Considerations Regarding the Need for Studies in Juvenile Animals

Considerations such as postnatal development and the utility of studies conducted using juvenile animals are discussed in this section.

A. Differences in Drug Safety Profiles between Mature and Immature Systems

Some therapeutics have shown different safety profiles in pediatric and adult patients. Inherent differences between mature and immature systems introduce the possibility of drug toxicity, or resistance to toxicity in immature systems that are not observed in mature systems. Several factors contribute to these potential differences. Postnatal growth and development can affect drug disposition and action. Examples include developmental changes in metabolism (including the maturation rate of Phase I and II enzyme activities), body composition (i.e., water and lipid partitions), receptor expression and function, growth rate, and organ functional capacity. These developmental processes are susceptible to modification or disruption by drugs.

Although some age-dependent effects can be largely predicted by knowledge of the changes in drug metabolic pathways during development, others cannot. There are several examples of drugs that exhibit differences in toxicity between adult and pediatric patients. These include the following:

- **Acetaminophen** — Acute acetaminophen toxicity is a classic example of how maturation can affect the toxicity profile of a drug. Young children are far less susceptible to acute acetaminophen toxicity than adults because children possess a higher rate of glutathione turnover and more active sulfation. Thus, they have a greater capacity to metabolize and detoxify an overdose of acetaminophen when compared to adults (Insel 1996).

- **Valproic acid** — In contrast to acetaminophen, young children treated with valproic acid appear disproportionately vulnerable to fatal hepatotoxicity (Dreifuss et al. 1987).

- **Chloramphenicol** — Chloramphenicol is associated with mortality in newborns because exposure is increased due to a longer half-life ($t_{½}$ = 26 h) compared to adults ($t_{½}$ = 4 h) (Kapusink-Uner et al. 1996).

- **Inhaled corticosteroids** — Inhaled corticosteroids have been found to decrease growth velocity in children, an irrelevant endpoint in adults (FDA Talk Paper, *Class Labeling for Intranasal and Orally Inhaled Corticosteroid Containing Drug Products Regarding the Potential for Growth Suppression in Children*, 1998).

- **Aspirin** — Aspirin should not be used to treat children with influenza or varicella infections because of their increased risk of developing Reye's syndrome, a complication not seen in adults (Belay et al. 1999).

- **Lamotrigine** — Children are at greater risk for developing hypersensitivity-type reactions, including Stevens-Johnson syndrome, when treated with lamotrigine (Guberman et al. 1999).

B. The Utility of Studies in Juvenile Animals

Adult clinical data can provide useful information regarding study design and dose selection for further study in children in some circumstances. Nonclinical developmental toxicity studies have traditionally focused on prenatal development, with only limited assessment of postnatal developmental effects. Animals used in multiple-dose toxicity studies are usually peripubertal. In some circumstances, data generated from these studies may provide sufficient information to support pediatric clinical trials without additional animal studies, particularly if the intended use includes adolescents but not younger children or infants. Since young animals in general exhibit developmental characteristics similar to pediatric patients, they are considered appropriate models for assessing drug effects in this population. The Agency believes that data from juvenile animal studies can contribute to the assessment of potential drug toxicity in the pediatric population, and can provide information that might not be derived from standard toxicology studies using adult animals, or safety information from adult humans.

It is thought that organ systems at highest risk for drug toxicity are those that undergo significant postnatal development. Thus, evaluation of postnatal developmental toxicity is a primary concern. The structural and functional characteristics of many organ systems differ significantly between children and adults as a result of the growth and development that takes place during postnatal maturation. Examples include the following:

- Brain, where neural development continues through adolescence (Rice and Barone 2000)
- Kidneys, where adult levels of function are first reached at approximately 1 year of age (Radde 1985)
- Lungs, where most alveolar maturation occurs in the first 2 years of life (Burri 1997)
- Immune system, where adult levels of IgG and IgA antibody responses are not achieved until about 5 and 12 years of age, respectively (Miyawaki et al. 1981)
- Reproductive system, where maturation is not completed until adolescence (Zoetis and Walls 2003)
- Skeletal system, where maturation continues well into adulthood for 25-30 years (Zoetis and Walls 2003)
- Gastrointestinal systems, which may have direct consequences on bioavailability, clearance, and biotransformation of drugs are functionally mature by about 1 year of age (Walthall 2005).

Studies in juvenile animals may be useful in the prediction of age-related toxicity in children, as shown in the following examples:

- The effects of phenobarbital on cognitive performance in children were predicted by experimental studies examining the effects of this drug on the developing rodent nervous system (Farwell et al. 1990; Fonseca et al. 1976; Diaz et al. 1977)
- The vulnerability of human neonates to hexachlorophene neurotoxicity was modeled in developing rats and monkeys (Towfighi 1980)
- The increased susceptibility of infants to verapamil-induced cardiovascular complications would be expected based on animal studies demonstrating a greater sensitivity of the immature heart to calcium channel blockade (Skovranek et al. 1986; Boucek et al. 1984)

- An increased risk of convulsions in young children treated with theophylline was predicted by studies of the preconvulsant effects of this agent in developing rodents (Mares et al. 1994; Yokoyama et al. 1997)

Examples of drug-induced postnatal developmental toxicity demonstrated in animals include the following:

- Neurobehavioral impairment in adult rats following early postnatal exposure to methamphetamine (Vorhees et al. 1994)
- The effects of methylphenidate on growth and endocrine function in young rats (Greeley and Kizer 1980; Pizzi et al. 1987)
- Apoptotic neurodegeneration in neonatal rats treated with NMDA receptor antagonists (Ikonomidou et al. 1999)
- Decreased myelination and axonal damage induced in preweanling rats by vigabatrin (Sidhu et al. 1997)
- Long-term changes in serotonergic innervation in rats exposed to fluoxetine during early juvenile life (Wegerer et al. 1999)
- Chondrotoxicity in immature animals treated with fluoroquinolones (Stahlmann et al. 1997)

Although the significance of these findings for humans is uncertain, there is evidence that some of these effects can be relevant to growing children, notably those of methylphenidate (Mattes and Gittelman 1983; Croche et al. 1979) and fluoroquinolones (Chang et al. 1996; Le Loet et al. 1991).

IV. General Considerations for Evaluation of Pharmaceuticals in Juvenile Animals

A. Scope of Nonclinical Safety Evaluation

The nonclinical safety evaluation of pediatric therapeutics should primarily focus on their potential effects on growth and development that have not been studied or identified in previous nonclinical and clinical studies. Juvenile animal testing may be useful in assessing potential developmental age-specific toxicities and differences in sensitivity between adult and immature animals. Although the toxicological assessment should focus primarily on the active moiety, testing the inactive ingredients in the clinical formulation can also be important, particularly when a drug's pharmacodynamics or distribution are altered by the inactive ingredients or when uncharacterized excipients are present. Additional recommendations on testing excipients can be found in the guidance for industry *Nonclinical Studies for the Safety Evaluation of Pharmaceutical Excipients.*[2] The toxicological assessment should include local and systemic analyses of effects on postnatal growth and development in the anticipated pediatric population. The known pharmacological and toxicological properties of the drug relative to the proposed patient population should be considered. Any concerns for postnatal developmental toxicity can be addressed either in juvenile animal studies or by modified study designs (e.g., modification of segment III reproductive toxicity studies to include animals of similar developmental status as the pediatric population of concern). Juvenile animal studies are especially relevant when a known target organ toxicity occurs in adults in tissues that undergo significant postnatal development. The extent and timing of nonclinical safety studies will depend on the available safety information for a particular product. For example, the information needed to support a new pediatric indication for an approved product used in adults may be quite different from the information needed to support pediatric use of a new molecular entity because of the postnatal developmental safety concerns in the later population. These concerns will be considered for their particular clinical indications on a case-by-case basis within the drug review divisions.

B. Timing of Juvenile Animal Studies in Relation to Clinical Testing

Specific recommendations regarding the timing of nonclinical toxicology studies are available in the ICH guidance for industry *M3 Nonclinical Safety Studies for the Conduct of Human Clinical Trials for Pharmaceuticals* (ICH M3 safety studies guidance). The recommendations presented here for juvenile animal studies may assist in identifying postnatal developmental toxicities that are not adequately assessed in general toxicity studies with mature animals and that may not be adequately and safely tested in pediatric clinical trials.

1. Long-Term Exposure in Pediatric Subjects

Most clinical studies in pediatric subjects do not involve long-term exposure to a therapy because they are generally of short-term duration (less than 6 months). This is especially true when the trials are intended to determine pharmacokinetics rather than efficacy. As a result, long-term exposure during postnatal developmental periods is not usually addressed in pediatric clinical trials. If the drug is indicated for chronic use then some assessment of the long-term developmental effects of the drug in animals should be made before marketing. However, in those cases when pediatric clinical studies do involve long-term exposure, we recommend conducting juvenile animal studies *before* initiation of the long-term clinical studies. When designing juvenile animal studies, the age of the pediatric population for which the drug is intended is important. Neonates, infants, and older children are at very different developmental stages, and appropriate nonclinical data should support the drug's use in the intended pediatric population.

2. Short-Term Exposure in Pediatric Subjects

Depending on the indication and use of the drug, safety concerns, and the number of subjects exposed, there may be a need for juvenile animal studies in conjunction with clinical studies even if the trials are designed for short-term exposure. Because juvenile animal studies may identify potential hazards and these hazards may have relevance to human safety, it may be more useful to complete juvenile animal studies before conducting clinical studies so that appropriate monitoring can be incorporated into the clinical trial design to limit human risk.

3. Insufficient Clinical Data to Support Initiation of Pediatric Studies

Typically, pediatric subjects are included in clinical trials after there has been considerable experience in the adult population. When there is insufficient clinical data or experience because of minimal prior adult and pediatric experience, completed juvenile animal studies are needed before initiation of pediatric clinical trials regardless of whether the clinical trials involve long-term exposures. Similarly, when there have been reports of adverse effects with off-label use in pediatric patients and there are inadequate data to evaluate the relationship between the drug and the adverse effects, completed juvenile animal studies are needed before initiation of pediatric clinical studies. The timing of juvenile animal studies relative to clinical testing of therapeutics indicated for serious or life-threatening pediatric conditions will be considered on a case-by-case basis by the review division.

C. Issues to Consider Regarding Juvenile Animal Studies

These considerations are important in determining the appropriateness and design of juvenile animal studies: (1) the intended or likely use of the drug in children; (2) the timing of dosing in relation to phases of growth and development in pediatric populations and juvenile animals; (3) the potential differences in pharmacological and toxicological profiles between mature and immature systems; and (4) any established temporal developmental differences in animals relative to pediatric populations. We also recommend that endpoints relevant to identifying target organ toxicity across species be included in the juvenile animal study design. Juveniles generally undergo more dynamic development than is seen in the relatively stable adult. Although the greatest concern is with chronic, long-term therapy, the duration of anticipated treatment of the pediatric population should be considered in relation to the duration of developmentally sensitive phases. For instance, a relatively short exposure time for neonates may cover a period of more substantial development than would a longer exposure in prepubescent children where development occurs over a much longer time frame. It is important for juvenile animal toxicology studies to be designed efficiently, using the least number of animals to identify potential pediatric safety concerns. Whenever feasible, we recommend designing an initial study to address endpoints of concern for multiple potential pediatric populations. In all cases, studies using juvenile animals are appropriate when adequate information cannot be generated using standard nonclinical studies or from clinical trials. The following issues are specific to studies in juvenile animals for assessing toxicity.

1. Developmental Stage of Intended Population

Consideration should be given to the age of the intended population and thus the stage of postnatal development. The condition to be treated may also influence the type, extent, and timing of testing considered appropriate. Selection of appropriate endpoints in the nonclinical studies to address concerns for the specific pediatric populations is important. Recommendations regarding specific age ranges of pediatric subpopulations are discussed in the ICH guidance for industry *E11 Clinical Investigation of Medicinal Products in the Pediatric Population.*

2. Evaluating Data to Determine When Juvenile Animal Studies Should Be Used

Evaluation of the available data is important when considering the need for studies in juvenile animals. Toxicity studies in juvenile animals may be appropriate when available nonclinical or clinical data are insufficient to support reasonable safety of a therapeutic for pediatric patients. Gaps in the age ranges of rodent and nonrodent species used in standard toxicity testing are widely acknowledged. These age gaps can affect assessment of nervous system toxicity endpoints in particular because of the extended process of maturation. Standard toxicity studies with adult animals cannot assess all of the relevant endpoints, especially growth present in the immature animal. In other circumstances, however, juvenile animal studies would be neither informative nor necessary. For example, juvenile animal studies might not be necessary when: (1) data from similar therapeutics in a class have identified a particular hazard and additional data are unlikely to change this perspective; (2) there are adequate clinical data and adverse events of concern have not been observed during clinical use; (3) target organ toxicity would not be expected to differ in sensitivity between adult and pediatric patients because the target organ of toxicity is functionally mature in the intended pediatric population and younger children with the functionally immature tissue are not expected to receive the drug.

Most drugs that are intended for use in pediatric patients have established efficacy and safety profiles in adult humans. Some data may also be available from pediatric patients aged 12 years or older. For some drugs a preponderance of clinical data will be obtained from children, as in the case of inhaled corticosteroids (FDA Talk Paper, *Class Labeling for Intranasal and Orally Inhaled Corticosteroid Containing Drug Products Regarding the Potential for Growth Suppression in Children,* 1998). For approved drugs that have already undergone extensive clinical testing, substantial nonclinical pharmacology and toxicology data will have already been performed. The toxicology assessment generally includes studies of general toxicity, reproductive toxicity, genetic toxicity, carcinogenicity, and special toxicities, as well as studies in juvenile animals, if available. Target organs of toxicity of the drug both in humans and animals should have been identified in these studies. A thorough evaluation of these data should enable scientists to: (1) judge the adequacy of the nonclinical information; (2) identify some of the potential safety concerns for the intended population; and (3) identify any gaps in the data that might be addressed by testing in juvenile animals.

3. Considering Developmental Windows When Determining Duration of Clinical Use

Based on the observation that embryo-fetal development is especially sensitive to perturbation during organogenesis, tissues that undergo significant postnatal development in pediatric patients and juvenile animals may also have greater sensitivity to certain drug-induced toxicities than mature tissues. Organ systems identified as undergoing considerable postnatal growth and development include the nervous, reproductive, pulmonary, renal, skeletal, gastrointestinal, hepatobiliary, and immune systems. Given the variable rate of postnatal development during different periods of childhood, the definition of long-term treatment can vary by pediatric population. Intended treatment of several weeks may not be considered long term in early adolescence, but might involve considerable development for the neonate given the duration of some developmental windows.

4. Timing of Exposure

The timing of the intended use of the drug as it relates to periods of rapid postnatal growth and development is important. If the drug is intended for use in children undergoing phases of rapid overall growth and development, it is important to evaluate an animal model undergoing a corresponding growth phase. Organ systems mature at specific times in specific species. Human-to-animal comparisons of developmental periods for the nervous, reproductive, skeletal, pulmonary, immune, renal, cardiac, and metabolic systems are presented in Section VII at the end of this guidance. These can be used as general guides to appropriate periods of treatment to assess the development of specific systems in various animal models. Immature animals have accelerated chronological development compared to humans, which can facilitate evaluation of long-term effects following acute or chronic exposure using well-defined endpoints (e.g., assessment of reproductive or nervous function).

5. Selection of Study Models

In addition to consideration of models and endpoint assessments based on the intended pediatric human use, target organs for toxicological and pharmacological activity identified in adults need special consideration. It is important that organ systems identified as specific targets of drug toxicity in adults and that undergo significant postnatal development be studied in juvenile animals for those specific effects, even when the primary postnatal developmental period in humans does not coincide with the intended treatment phase. This is based on the observation that development is generally a continuous event. Additionally, a therapeutic target tissue may be developmentally regulated by other tissues or organ systems. In such cases, it may be advisable to examine the effects of the drug during the stages of development relevant to all of those tissues/organs in a test species.

V. General Considerations in Designing Toxicity Studies in Juvenile Animals

A. Types of Studies

Testing approaches can use generalized screening tests to provide hazard identification or can be designed to specifically address identified concerns. We recommend the selection of an appropriate, scientifically justified study design. The effects of dosing and handling on immature animals can be systematically assessed. Studies conducted in juvenile animals to support the safety of pediatric therapeutics may either be protocols designed to address a specific safety concern, or modified peri- and postnatal developmental study protocols. Dedicated juvenile animal protocols can be designed to address specific concerns based on known properties of the drug, product class, or other information. Modified repeat-dose toxicity studies can provide a more general screen for potential hazards in some instances. However, we recommend that such studies modify the animal age at study initiation, duration of treatment, and endpoints assessed to address the specific concerns. Modification of standard ICH studies designed to address developmental stages C-F[3] would include ensuring adequate exposure in juvenile animals during the postnatal period and assessment of developmental endpoints appropriate for the intended pediatric population. Assessment of developmental endpoints not usually included in standard repeat-dose toxicity studies also may be appropriate. In addition to ensuring adequate exposure to the drug, histopathologic examinations and effects on specific growth parameters and functionally immature tissues in the juvenile animal would be important. In these modified designs dosing can be initiated with animals younger than usual and extended until the developmental period for the intended pediatric population has been completed in the animal species in accordance with the age of the pediatric patients who would use the drug. Information from such studies can be compared with the findings from treated adults of the same species to evaluate whether the effects are specific to juvenile animals.

B. Animals

1. Species

The species of the juvenile animal tested should be appropriate for evaluating toxicity endpoints important for the intended pediatric population. Traditionally, rats and dogs have been the rodent and nonrodent species of choice. In some circumstances, however, other species may be more appropriate. For example, when drug metabolism in a particular species differs significantly from humans, an alternative species (e.g., minipigs, pigs, monkeys) may be more appropriate for testing. When determining an appropriate species, sponsors are encouraged to consider certain factors, such as the following:

- Pharmacology, pharmacokinetics, and toxicology of the therapeutic agent
- Comparative developmental status of the major organs of concern between juvenile animals and pediatric patients
- Sensitivity of the selected species to a particular toxicity

A study in juveniles from one animal species may be sufficient to evaluate toxicity endpoints for therapeutics that are well characterized in both adult humans and animals. It is anticipated that this evaluation often can be accomplished in the rodent using modified perinatal and postnatal developmental studies, although other approaches can be used.

2. Age

The age of the animals at initiation of dosing should be determined by the postnatal development parameters of interest. It is important that the stage of development in the animals being studied be comparable to that in the intended pediatric population.

3. Sex and Sample Size

We recommend including both male and female animals in these studies. It is important that adequate numbers of animals are used to demonstrate the presence or absence of effects of the test substance. When determining the sample size, consideration of the magnitude of the biologic effect that is of concern is also important. The particular study design used (e.g., a screening study or one designed to address an identified concern, modification of a standard design, composite or split litter design) will influence the number of animals it takes for an adequate evaluation.

C. Exposure

1. Route of Administration and Dosage Formulation

When performing nonclinical studies, the intended clinical route of administration and dosage formulation[4] should be used unless an alternate route of administration and dosage formulation provides greater exposure or is less invasive with adequate exposure. Assessment of toxic effects by more than one route of administration can be appropriate if the drug is intended for clinical use by more than one route of administration. When different routes are expected to result in differences in systemic and local exposure of such magnitude that occurrence of postnatal toxicity would be expected, sponsors should consider testing by multiple routes. When the intended clinical administration is intravenous, this route should be sufficient. Since the primary purpose of these studies is to identify potential hazards, small changes in exposure/distribution by route generally would not be considered important.

Since adverse effects can sometimes be related to metabolic differences between adult and juvenile animals, toxicokinetic studies can provide useful information for assisting in study interpretation. Assessment of developmental differences in parent drug disposition and profiles of significant metabolites in juvenile animals should be made according to established guidelines (see the ICH guideline for industry *S3A Toxicokinetics: Assessment of Systemic Exposure in Toxicity Studies*).

2. Frequency and Duration of Exposure

The frequency of administration should be relevant to the intended clinical use of the drug. In some cases, however, the use of dosing frequencies similar to those anticipated for clinical administration are not feasible because of technical considerations for the animal models used. Changes in frequency can be made when variables such as metabolic and kinetic differences are considered.

The duration of treatment in animals should include at least the significant periods of relevant postnatal development for the selected species. When the aim of the study is to evaluate potential long-term effects, dosing duration should be increased relative to the intended therapeutic use. One approach to consider is establishing exposure and initial tolerability in a dose-range finding study followed by a definitive study powered to assess specific concerns. Treatment-free periods designed to assess reversibility of possible adverse effects should also be considered. Inclusion of recovery periods in studies can be valuable in distinguishing acute to intermediate pharmacodynamic effects from frank developmental toxicity, and this information could influence the evaluation of potential human risk. Depending on the concern being addressed, it may be sufficient to assess delayed toxicity through organ maturity or it may be necessary to continue until the juvenile animal reaches adulthood.

3. Dose Selection

It is important to establish a clear dose-response relationship for adverse effects in juvenile animals, when possible. The high dose should produce identifiable toxicity (either developmental or general). The intermediate dose should produce some toxicity so that a dose-response relationship can be demonstrated if one exists. The low dose should produce little or no toxicity, and a NOAEL should be identified, if possible. We recommend evaluating and potentially modifying intermediate and low doses in relation to those that produce the desired pharmacodynamic effect in the test species.

D. Toxicological Endpoints and Timing of Monitoring

The selection of toxicological endpoints to be monitored in a juvenile animal study is critical for assessing the effects of a drug on development and growth. Designing studies to determine drug effects on overall postnatal growth as well as postnatal development of specific organ systems (e.g., skeletal, renal, lung, nervous, immunologic, cardiovascular, and reproductive) is appropriate. It is important that studies include measurement of overall growth (e.g., body weight, growth velocity per unit time, tibial length), clinical observations, measurement of organ weights, gross and microscopic examinations, assessment of sexual maturation (mating, fertility), and neurobehavioral testing. More specific measurements can be reserved for case-specific evaluations based on the knowledge of the pharmacologic or toxicologic target. Clinical pathology determinations can also be useful but can be limited by the technical feasibility of obtaining adequate samples for analysis, particularly in the case of rodents. For developmental neurotoxicity assessments, well-established methods should be used to monitor key central nervous system (CNS) functions, including assessments of reflex ontogeny, sensorimotor function, locomotor activity, reactivity, learning, and memory. Modifications of existing toxicity designs or *de novo* juvenile studies should be used depending on the concerns to be addressed.

It can be helpful to determine the relationship between toxicologic endpoints and drug exposure (e.g., predosing, immediately postdosing, time of peak plasma concentration). To differentiate long-term effects on development from acute effects, it might be appropriate to measure certain endpoints immediately before daily administration of the drug. Also, adding recovery group animals is helpful in determining whether the drug-induced effects are reversible. The more specific the concern, the more directed the study design approach can be. A more generalized screening approach may be useful if little information is available.

VI. General Considerations for Application of Juvenile Animal Data in Risk Management

A. Use in Clinical Trials

It is important that nonclinical toxicology studies designed to support the safety of clinical trials in pediatric subjects identify hazards specific to the treated population. These studies can provide information useful in limiting the risk of experiencing adverse events and identify appropriate clinical monitoring. When adverse effects are observed in nonclinical toxicology studies, there are a number of possible uses of these findings. Biomarkers of adverse effects could be identified in nonclinical studies that would be useful in monitoring subjects in clinical trials. In cases where biomarkers cannot be identified or safely used in clinical studies, nonclinical pharmacokinetic data could be useful because a given adverse effect would be associated with a particular level of systemic exposure which might be extrapolated to clinical use. Blood level monitoring could then be used in clinical trials to minimize the probability of such an adverse effect occurring. If toxicities identified in juvenile animal studies are likely to occur in pediatric patients, cannot be monitored clinically, and would not be considered an acceptable potential consequence of exposure, it may not be possible to safely conduct pediatric clinical trials. Consideration of the risk-benefit analysis of a given drug therapy is important.

B. Use in Product Approval

Nonclinical toxicology studies in juvenile animal models could demonstrate adverse effects that should be considered in seeking postmarketing commitments by the sponsor, in labeling a product for pediatric use, or in determining the approvability of a drug for pediatric use. Delayed or irreversible adverse effects might be identified in animal studies but not in clinical trials because the pediatric clinical trial might have been of insufficient duration to demonstrate the adverse effect. It is possible that biomarkers of adverse effects could be identified in nonclinical studies that were not seen in clinical trials, but might nevertheless be important to include in the product label. Depending on the nature and severity of these adverse effects and the risk-benefit relationship of the intended use, the sponsor might conduct long-term follow-up human safety studies as a postmarketing commitment. The sponsor might conduct long-term follow-up studies even following acute drug exposure if these effects were found to be delayed or irreversible. Use of the drug could be restricted to serious indications based on nonclinical findings even if the adverse effects were not demonstrated in clinical trials. In this case, the product label would include information on the relevant adverse effects observed in nonclinical studies. Adverse effects associated with chronic drug exposure in nonclinical studies might not have been observed in clinical trials of comparable length. In such a case, the label might be written to reflect these findings. Juvenile animal studies might also be useful in identifying specific age groups in which the drug should not be used or in determining unsafe parameters of exposure. Finally, it is possible that nonclinical findings could result in a product label that specifically warns against use in pediatric patients based on a risk-benefit analysis.

VII. Human-to-Animal Comparisons of Developmental Periods

The information on comparative developmental timing, shown in Tables 1 – 8, was considered current at the time this guidance was developed. These comparisons should be considered with new information as it becomes available in deciding how best to design appropriate juvenile animal studies to address risks to the pediatric population. Neither the human nor the animal data represent a precise determination of the timelines of development due to the inherent variability and different endpoints examined. Because of the nature of science, these tables should only serve as a general starting point.

Table 1. Nervous System

Developmental Event	Postnatal Developmental Period			
	Human (Years)	Primate (Weeks)	Dog (Weeks)	Rat (Days)
Glutamate receptors[1] (Maximal binding)	1-2 Cortex Decline to adult 2-16			28 Decline to adult >28

Table 1. (Continued)

Developmental Event	Postnatal Developmental Period			
Monoamine system[2]	2-4 Maximum receptor density			21-30 Adult levels
Ocular dominance3	0-3			21-35
Cerebellum persistent external germinal layer[3]	0.6-2			0-21
Rapid phase of myelination ends[4]	2			25-30
Cognitive development Delayed response learning[5]	1-2	9-36	12-16	10-35

[1] Ikonomidou et al. 1999

[2] Rice and Barone 2000

[3] Sidhu et al. 1997; Kimmel and Buelke-Sam 1994

[4] Radde 1985

[5] Wood et al. 2004

Table 2. Reproductive System

Developmental Event	Postnatal Developmental Period				
	Human (Years)	Rhesus Monkey (Years)	Dog (Days)	Mouse (Days)	Rat (Days)
Puberty[1]	11-12	2.5-3	180-240	35-45	40-60

[1] DeSesso and Harris 1995; Marty et al. 2003; Beckman and Feuston 2003; Lewis et al. 2002

Table 3. Skeletal System

Developmenta l Event	Postnatal Developmental Period					
Fusion of 2° Ossification Centers[1]	Human (Years)	Monkey (Years)	Dog (Years)	Rabbit (Weeks)	Rat (Weeks)	Mouse (Weeks)
Femur Distal Epiphysis	14-19	3-6	0.7-0.9	32	15-162	12-13

[1] Zoetis 2003

Table 4. Pulmonary System[1]

Developmental Event	Postnatal Developmental Period (Days)		
Alveoli Formation[2,3,4]	**Human**	**Rat**	**Mouse**
Onset	Prenatal	1-4	1-2
Completion	730	28	28

[1] The stages of lung development (glandular, canalicular, saccular, alveolar) at birth varies with the species. Human lungs have few alveoli and are considered in the alveolar stage at birth. Rodent lungs are less developed and considered in the saccular stage without alveoli at birth (Zoetis and Hurtt 2003).

[2] Burri 1997

[3] Merkus et al. 1996

[4] Tschanz and Burri 1997

Table 5. Immune System

Developmental Event	Postnatal Developmental Period (Days)	
	Human	**Mice**
B-cell Development[1]	Prenatal	Prenatal
T-cell Development[1]	Prenatal	Prenatal
NK-cell Development[1]	Prenatal	21
T-dependent Antibody response[1]	0	14 41-56 Adult level
T-independent Antibody response[1]	45-90	0 14-21 Adult level
Adult level IgG[1]	1825	42-56

[1] Holladay and Smialowicz 2000

Table 6a. Renal — Functional

Developmental Event	Postnatal Developmental Period (Days)	
	Human	**Rat**
Glomerulo-/Nephrogenesis[1,2]	Prenatal	8-14
Adult GFR and tubular secretion[1,2]	45-180	15-21

[1] Snodgrass 1992

[2] Travis 1991

Table 6b. Renal — Anatomical

Developmental Event	Postnatal Developmental Period (Weeks)					
	Human	Dog	Rabbit	Rat	Mouse	Pig
Completion of Nephrogenesis[1]	Prenatal Week 35	2	2-3	4-6	Prenatal	3

[1] Zoetis 2003

Table 7. Metabolism

Developmental Modulation of Phase I/II Metabolism			
	Maturation of Enzyme Activity		
Enzyme	Human (Years)	Rat (Days)	Rabbit (Days)
CYP2D6[1,2]	0-3	NA*	NA*
CYP2E1[2,3,4]	0-1	4-17 ↓ Post weaning male>female	14-35 2X adult @35
CYP1A2[1,5,6,7]	0.5 1(> adult)	7-100 Low levels	21-60
CYP2C8[1,2]	<1	NA*	NA*
CYP2C9[1,2]	<0.5 0.5 (> adult)	NA*	NA*
CYP3A4[2]	0-2	NA*	NA*
Acetylation[1,2]	1 (35% adult)	NA*	NA*
Methylation[1,2]	<1 (50% adult)	NA*	NA*
Glucuronidation[1,2]	0 (>adult) 12		NA*
Sulfation[1,2]	0	NA*	NA*

* NA = not available

[1] Kearns and Reed 1989

[2] Leeder and Kerns 1997

[3] Waxman, Morrissey, Le Balnc 1989

[4] Peng, Porter, Ding, Coon 1991

[5] Ding, Peng, Coon 1992

[6] Imaoka, Fujita, Funai 1991

[7] Pineau, Daujatz, Pichard, Girard, Angevain 1991

Table 8. Cardiac[1]

Cardiac Parameter		Postnatal Developmental Period (Maturation Level Similar to Adult)	
	Human (Years)	Dog	Rat (Weeks)
Electrophysiolog y (ECG)	5-7 years	NA*	3-8
Cardiac Output (CO) and Hemodynamics	Birth 138 bpm; Adults 85 bpm. <2 yrs: Smaller ventricular vol., stroke index, ejection fraction vs. adult Birth BP 62/40; 2 months 85/47; 0.5-8 yrs. Diastolic 58-62	Increase in BP and decrease in HR from 1 week to 0.5 years	Early increase in HR then constant into adulthood High CO and low PVR Neonate-puberty systolic BP doubles reaches maturity by 10 weeks
Myocytes	Diploid at birth compared to 60% in adults (40% polyploidy)	NA*	Primarily diploid in infant and adult
Coronary Vasculature	Diameter of arteries doubled at 1 yr. max at 30 yrs. Capillary angiogenesis occurs postnatally and density decreases with age	Capillary angiogenesis occurs postnatally and density decreases with age	Capillary angiogenesis occurs postnatally arterial maturation by 1 month
Cardiac innervation	Neuron number increase and reach adult pattern/density in childhood	Continued development during 2-4 months	Adrenergic pattern mature by 3 weeks and nerve den-sity mature by 5 weeks. Cholinergic matures postnatally

* NA = not available

[1] Hew and Keller 2003

References

Beckman, DA. & Feuston, M. 2003, Landmarks in the Development of the Female Reproductive System, Birth Defects Research, (part B), 68,137-143.

Belay, ED; Bresee, JS; Holman, RC; Khan, AS; Shahriari, A; et al., 1999, Reye's Syndrome in the United States from 1981 through 1997, N Engl *J Med*, 340,1377-1382.

Boucek Jr. RJ; Shelton, M; Artman, M; Mushlin, PS; Starnes, VA; et al., 1984, Comparative Effects of Verapamil, Nifedipine, and Diltiazem on Contractile Function in the Isolated Immature and Adult Rabbit Heart, *Pediatric Res*, 18,948-952.

Burri, P. 1997, Structural Aspects of Prenatal and Postnatal Development and Growth of the Lung, Lung Growth and Development, Ed. JA McNoald, Marcel Dekker, Inc., New York, p. 1- 35.

Chang, H; Chung, MH. & Kim, JH. 1996, Pefloxacin-Induced Arthropathy in an Adolescent with Brain Abscess, *Scand J Infect Dis*, 28,641-643.

Committee on Drugs, 1995, American Academy of Pediatrics, Guidelines for the Ethical Conduct of Studies to Evaluate Drugs in Pediatric Populations, *Pediatrics*, 95(2) 286-294.

Croche, AF; Lipman, RS; Overall, JE. & Hung, W. 1979, The Effects of Stimulant Medication on the Growth of Hyperkinetic Children, *Pediatrics*, 63(6),847-50.

DeSesso, JM. & Harris, SB. 1995, Principles Underlying Developmental Toxicity, Toxicology Risk Assessment, Eds. A Fan and LW Cgabg, Marcel Dekker, New York.

Diaz, J; Schain, RJ. & Bailey, BG. 1977, Phenobarbital-Induced Brain Growth Retardation in Artificially Reared Rat Pups, *Biol Neonate*, 32,77-82.

Ding, X, Peng, HM. & Coon, MF. 1992, Cytochromes P450 NMa, NMb (2G1) and LM4 (1A2) are Differentially Expressed During Development in Rabbit Olfactory Mucosa and Liver, *Mol Pharmacol*, 42(N6),1027-1032.

Division of Pulmonary Drug Products, 1998, *Class Labeling for Intranasal and Oral Inhaled Corticosteroids Containing Drug Products Regarding the Potential for Growth Suppression in Children*, Center for Drug Evaluation and Research, the Food and Drug Administration, http://www.fda.gov/cder/news/cs-label.htm.

Dreifuss, FE; Santilli, N; Langer, DH; Sweeney, KP; Moline, KA. et al., 1987, Valproic Acid Hepatic Fatalities: A Retrospective Review, *Neurology*, 37, 379-385.

Farwell, JR; Lee, YJ; Hirtz, DG; Sulzbacher, SI; Ellenberg, JH. et al., 1990, Phenobarbital for Febrile Seizures — Effects on Intelligence and on Seizure Recurrence, N Engl *J Med*, 322,364-369.

FDA Talk Paper, November 9, 1998, Class Labeling for Intranasal and Orally Inhaled Corticosteroid Containing Drug Products Regarding the Potential for Growth Suppression in Children.

FDAMA, 1997, Pub. L., 105-115, 21 U.S.C.

FDAMA, January 3, 2001, Pub. S.1789, Best Pharmaceuticals for Children Act.

Fonseca, NM; Sell, AB. & Carlini, EA. 1976, Differential Behavioral Responses of Male and Female Adult Rats Treated with Five Psychotropic Drugs in the Neonatal Stage, *Psychopharmacologia*, 46,253-268.

Greely, GH. & Kizer, JS. 1980, The Effects of Chronic Methylphenidate Treatment on Growth and Endocrine Function in the Developing Rat, *J Pharmacol Exp Ther*, 215,545-551.

Guberman, AH; Besag, FM; Brodie, MJ; Dooley, JM; Duchowny, MS et al., 1999, Lamotrigine-Associated Rash: Risk/Benefit Considerations in Adults and Children, *Epilepsia*, 40,985-991.

Hew, KW. & Keller, KA. 2003, *Postnatal Anatomical and Functional Development of the Heart: A Species Comparison*, Birth Defects Research, (part B), 68,309-320.

Holladay, SD. & Smialowicz, R. 2000, Development of the Murine and Human Immune System: Different Effects of Immunotoxicants Depend on Time of Exposure, *Environ Health Perspect*, 108,463-473.

Hong, J; Pan, J; Dong, Z; Ning, SM. & Yang, CS. 1987, Regulation of N-Nitrosodimethylamine Demethylase in Rat Liver and Kidney, *Cancer Res*, 47(N11),5948-5953.

Ikonomidou, C; Bosch, F; Miksa, M; Bittigau, P; Vockler, J; Dikranian, K. et al., 1999, Blockade of NMDA Receptors and Apoptotic Neurodegeneration in the Developing Brain, *Science*, 283,70-74.

Imaoka, S; Fujita, S. & Funae, Y. 1991, Age Dependent Expression of Cytochrome P450s in Rat Liver, *Biochem Biophys Acta*, 1097(N3),187-192.

Insel, PA; 1996, *Analgesic-Antipyretic and Antiinflammatory Agents, Goodman & Gilman's The Pharmacological Basis of Therapeutics*, 9th ed., Ed. JG Hardman, LE Limbird, PB Molinoff, RW Ruddon, and AG Gilman, McGraw-Hill, New York, p.632.

Kapusnik-Uner, JE; Sande, MA. & Chambers, HF. 1996, *Antimicrobial Agents, Goodman & Gilman's The Pharmacological Basis of Therapeutics*, 9th ed., Ed. JG Hardman, LE Limbird, PB Molinoff, RW Ruddon, and AG Gilman, McGraw-Hill, New York, p.1124-1153.

Kearns, LK & Reed, MD 1989, Clinical Pharmacokinetics in Infants and Children. A Reappraisal, *Clin Pharmacokin*, 17(supp 1),29-67.

Kimmel, CA, Kavlock, RJ. & Francis, EZ. 1992, Animal Models for Assessing Developmental Toxicity, Similarities and Differences Between Children and Adults, Implications for Risk Assessment, Ed. PS Guzelian, CJ Henry, and SS Olin, ILSI press, Washington DC.

Kimmel, CA. & Buelke-Sam, J; 1994, Target Organ Toxicology Series, Ed. Taylor and Frances, Raven Press.

Langston, C; Kida, K; Reed, M. & Thurlbeck, WM. 1984, Human Lung Growth in Late Gestation and in the Neonate, The American Review of Respiratory Disease, 129,607-613.

Lauffman, RE. 1994, Scientific Issues in Biomedical Research, *In: Children as Research Subjects, Ed. MA Grodin and LH Glantz*, Oxford University Press, Oxford, England, p. 1-17.

Le Loet, X; Fessard, C; Noblet, C; Sait, LA. & Moore, N. 1991, Severe Polyarthropathy in an Adolescent Treated with Pefloxacin, *J. Rheumatology*, 18,1941-1942.

Leeder, JS. & Kearns, GL. 1997, *Pharmacogenetics in Pediatrics: Implications for Practice, New Frontiers in Pediatric Drug Therapy*, Pediatric Clinics of North America, 44(1),55-77.

Lewis, EM; Barnett Jr., JF; Freshwater, L; Hoberman, AM. & Christian, MS. 2002, Sexual Maturation Data for CRL Sprague-Dawley Rats: Criteria and Confounding Factors, *Drug and Chemical Toxicology*, 25(4),437-458.

Lovejoy, FH. 1982, Fatal Benzyl Alcohol Poisoning in Neonatal Intensive Care Units, *Am J Dis Child*, 136,974-975.

Mares, P; Kubova, H. & Czuczwar, SJ. 1994, Aminophylline Exhibits Convulsant Action in Rats During Ontogenesis, *Brain Development*, 16(4),296-300.

Marty, MS; Chapin, R; Parks, L. & Thorsrud, B. 2003, *Development and Maturation of the Male Reproductive System*, Birth Defects Research, (part B), 68,125-136.

Mattes, JA. & Gittelman, R. 1983, Growth of Hyperactive Children on Maintenance Regimen of Methylphenidate, *Arch Gen Psychiatry*, 40,317-321.

Merkus PJFM et al., 1996, Human Lung Growth: A Review, *Pediatric Pulmonol*, 21, 383-397.

Miyawaki, T; Moriya, N; Nagaoki, T. & Taniguchi, N. 1981, Maturation of B-Cell Differentiation Ability and T-Cell Regulatory Function in Infancy and Childhood, *Immunol Rev*, 57,61-87.

Peng, HM; Porter, TD & Ding, XX. & Coon, MJ. 1991, Differences in the Developmental Expression of Rabbit Cytochromes P450 2E1 and 2E2, *Mol Pharmacol*, 40(N1),58-62.

Pineau, T; Daujat, M; Pichard, L; Girard, F; Angevain, J; et al., 1991, Developmental Expression of Rabbit Cytochrome P450 CYP1A1, CYP1A2, CYP3A6 Genes, Effect of Weaning and Rifampicin, *Cur J Biochem*, 197(N1),145-153.

Pizzi, WJ; Rode, EC. & Barnhart, JE. 1987, Differential Effects of Methylphenidate on the Growth of Neonatal and Adolescent Rats, *Neurotox Teratol*, 9,107-111.

Radde, IC, 1985, Mechanism of Drug Absorption and Their Development, *Textbook of Pediatric Clinical Pharmacology*, Ed. SM Macleod and IC Radde, PSG Publishing Co., Littleton, MA. p. 17-43.

Rice, D. & Barone Jr., S. 2000, Critical Periods of Vulnerability for the Developing Nervous System: Evidence from Humans and Animal Models, *Environ Health Persp*, 108(Suppl. 3) 511-533.

Rodier, PM; Cohen, IR. & Buelke-Sam, J. 1994, *Developmental Neurotoxicology, Developmental Toxicology*, 2nd ed., Ed. CA Kimmel and J Buelke-Sam, Raven Press, New York.

Sidhu, RS; Bigio, MR Del; Tuor, UI. & Seshia, SS. 1997, Low-Dose Vigabatrin (gamma-vinyl GABA)-Induced Damage in the Immature Rat Brain, *Exp Neurol*, 144,400-405.

Skovranek, J; Ostadal, B; Pelouch, V. & Prochazka, J. 1986, Ontogenetic Differences in Cardiac Sensitivity to Verapamil in Rats, *Pediatric Cardiol*, 7,25-29.

Snodgrass, WR. 1992, *Physiological and Biochemical Differences Between Children and Adults as Determinants of Toxic Response to Environmental Pollutants*, Similarities and Differences Between Children and Adults, Implications for Risk Assessment, Ed. PS Guzelian, CJ Henry, and SS Olin, ILSI press, Washington DC, p. 35-42.

Stahlmann, R; Chahoud, I; Thiel, R; Klug, S. & Forster, C. 1997, The Developmental Toxicity of Three Antimicrobial Agents Observed Only in Nonroutine Animal Studies, *Reprod Toxicol*, 11,1-7.

The 1998 Pediatric Rule, Regulations Requiring Manufacturers to Assess the Safety and Effectiveness of New Drugs and Biological Products in Pediatric Patients; Final Rule, 1998, *Fed Reg*, 63(231),66632 – 66672.

The List, 1998, List of Approved Drugs for Which Additional Pediatric Information May Produce Health Benefits in the Pediatric Population, *Fed Reg*, 63(97),27733.

Thurlbeck, WM, 1975, Postnatal Growth and Development of the Lung, *American Review of Respiratory Disease, 111*,804-804.

Towfighi, 1980, Experimental and Clinical Neurotoxicology, Spencer and Scaumburg, Eds., pp. 440-455, Williams and Williams, Baltimore.

Travis, LB. 1991, The Kidney and Urinary Tract Morphogenic Development and Anatomy, Rudolph's Pediatrics, 19th Ed., Chapter 25, pp. 1223-1236.

Tschanz, SA. & Burri, PH. 1997, Postnatal Lung Development and Its Impairment by Glucocorticoids, *Pediat Pulmonol*, Supp 16,247-249.

Vorhees, CV; Ahrens, KG; Acuff-Smith, KD; Schilling, MA. & Fisher, JE. 1994, Methamphetamine Exposure During Early Postnatal Development in Rats: I.

Acoustic Startle Augmentation and Spatial Learning Deficits, *Psychopharmacol*, 114,392-401.

Walthall, K; Cappon, GD; Hurtt, ME. & Zoetis, T. 2005, Postnatal Development of the Gastrointestinal System: A Species Comparison, Birth Defects Research, (part B), 74,132-156.

Waxman, DJ; Morrissey, JJ. & Le Balnc, GA. 1989, Female Predominant Rat Hepatic P450 Forms (IIE1) and 3(IIA1) Are Under Hormonal Regulatory Controls Distinct from Those of Sex Specific P450 Forms, *Endocrinology*, 270(N2), 458-471.

Wegerer, V; Moll, GH; Bagli, M; Rothenberger, A; Ruther, E; Huether, G; 1999, Persistently Increased Density of Serotonin Transporters in the Frontal Cortex of Rats Treated with Fluoxetine During Early Juvenile Life, *J Child Adolesc Psychopharmacol*, 9,13-24.

Wettrell, G. & Andersson, KE. 1986, Cardiovascular Drug II: Digioxin, Ther Drug Monitoring, 8,129-139.

Wood, SL; Beyer, BK. & Cappon, GD. 2004, Species Comparison of Postnatal CNS Development: Functional Measures, Birth Defects Research (in press).

Yokoyama, H; Onodera, K; Yagi, T. & Iinuma, K. 1997, Therapeutic Doses of Theophylline Exert Proconvulsant Effects in Developing Mice, *Brain Dev*, 19,403-407.

Zoetis, T. & Hurtt, ME. 2003, Species Comparison of Lung Development, Birth Defects Research, (part B), 68,121-124.

Zoetis, T; Tassinari, MS; Bagi, C; Walthall, K. & Hurtt, ME. 2003, *Species Comparison of Postnatal Bone Growth and Development,* Birth Defects Research, (part B), 68,86-110.

Zoetis, T. & Walls, I. 2003, *Principles and Practices for Direct Dosing of Pre-Weaning Mammals in Toxicity Testing and Research*, ILSI press, Washington DC, p.11 and p.13.

Zoetis, T. 2003, *Species Comparison of Anatomical and Functional Renal Development*, Birth Defects Research, (part B), 68,111-120.

End Notes

[1] This guidance has been prepared by the Pediatric Subcommittee to the Pharmacology and Toxicology Coordinating Committee within the Office of New Drugs (OND) in the Center for Drug Evaluation and Research (CDER) at the Food and Drug Administration. It does not apply to pediatric products regulated by the Center for Biologics Evaluation and Research (CBER). For information on products regulated by CBER, contact the appropriate CBER office.

[2] We update guidances periodically. To make sure you have the most recent version of a guidance, check the CDER guidance Web page at http://www.fda.gov/cder/guidance/index.htm.

[3] ICH guidance for industry *S5A Detection of Toxicity to Reproduction for Medicinal Products*

[4] We recommend safety evaluations of inactive ingredients be conducted to determine potential adverse effects in pediatric subjects. The type of testing is dependent on the extent to which this information is already well understood.

In: Safety Efforts in Pediatric Drug Development ISBN: 978-1-60741-565-7
Editor: Conor D. Byrne

Chapter 3

PEDIATRIC DRUG RESEARCH: STUDIES CONDUCTED UNDER BEST PHARMACEUTICALS FOR CHILDREN ACT

GAO

WHY GAO DID THIS STUDY

About two-thirds of drugs that are prescribed for children have not been studied and labeled for pediatric use, which places children at risk of being exposed to ineffective treatment or incorrect dosing. The Best Pharmaceuticals for Children Act (BPCA), enacted in 2002, encourages the manufacturers, or sponsors, of drugs that still have marketing exclusivity—that is, are on-patent—to conduct pediatric drug studies, as requested by the Food and Drug Administration (FDA). If they do so, FDA may extend for 6 months the period during which no equivalent generic drugs can be marketed. This is referred to as pediatric exclusivity.

BPCA required that GAO assess the effect of BPCA on pediatric drug studies and labeling. As discussed with the committees of jurisdiction, GAO (1) assessed the extent to which pediatric drug studies were being conducted under BPCA for on-patent drugs, including when drug sponsors declined to conduct the studies; (2) evaluated the impact of BPCA on labeling drugs for pediatric use and the process by which the labeling was changed; and (3) illustrated the range of diseases treated by the drugs studied under BPCA. GAO examined data about the drugs for which FDA requested studies under BPCA from 2002 through 2005. GAO also interviewed officials from relevant federal agencies, pharmaceutical industry representatives, and health advocates.

www.gao.gov/cgi-bin/getrpt?GAO-07-557.

To view the full product, including the scope and methodology, click on the link above. For more information, contact Marcia Crosse at (202) 512-7119 or crossem@gao.gov.

What GAO Found

Drug sponsors have initiated pediatric drug studies for most of the on-patent drugs for which FDA has requested studies, but no drugs were being studied when drug sponsors declined these requests. Sponsors agreed to 173 of the 214 written requests for pediatric studies of on-patent drugs. In cases where drug sponsors decline to study the drugs, BPCA provides for FDA to refer the study of these drugs to the Foundation for the National Institutes of Health (FNIH), a nonprofit corporation. FNIH had not funded studies for any of the nine drugs that FDA referred as of December 2005.

Most drugs (about 87 percent) granted pediatric exclusivity under BPCA had labeling changes—often because the pediatric drug studies found that children may have been exposed to ineffective drugs, ineffective dosing, overdosing, or previously unknown side effects. However the process for approving labeling changes was often lengthy. It took from 238 to 1,055 days for information to be reviewed and labeling changes to be approved for 18 drugs (about 40 percent), and 7 of those took more than 1 year. Drugs were studied under BPCA for the treatment of a wide range of diseases, including those that are common, serious, or life threatening to children. These drugs represented more than 17 broad categories of disease, such as cancer.

The Department of Health and Human Services stated that the report provides a significant amount of data and analysis and generally explains the BPCA process, but expressed concern that it did not sufficiently acknowledge the success of BPCA or clearly describe some elements of FDA's process. GAO incorporated comments as appropriate.

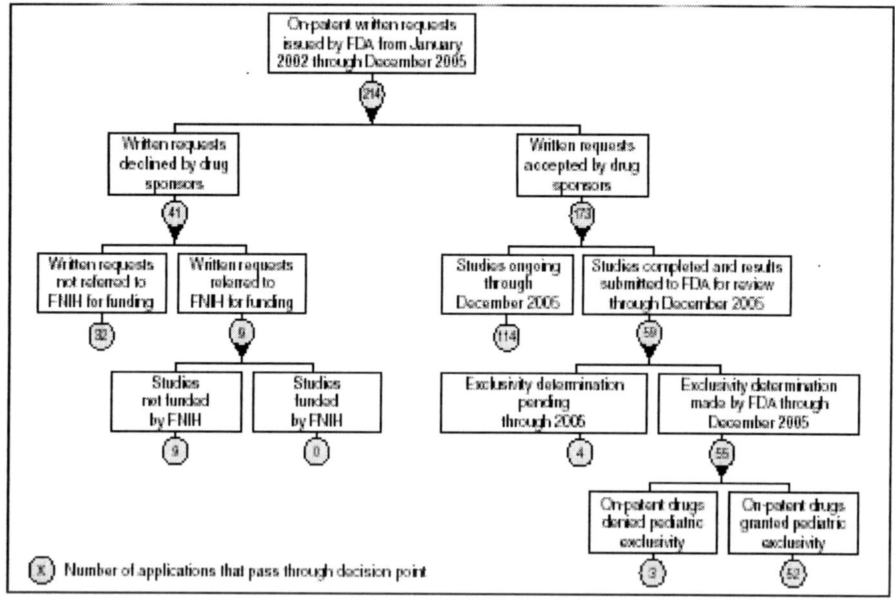

Source: GAO.

Written Requests Issued under BPCA for the Study of On-Patent Drugs (2002-2005)

ABBREVIATIONS

BPCA	Best Pharmaceuticals for Children Act
FDA	Food and Drug Administration
FDAMA	Food and Drug Administration Modernization Act of 1997
FNIH	Foundation for the National Institutes of Health
HHS	Department of Health and Human Services
HIV	Human Immunodeficiency Virus
NDDI	Newborn Drug Development Initiative
NIH	National Institutes of Health

March 22, 2007

The Honorable Edward M. Kennedy
Chairman
The Honorable Michael B. Enzi
Ranking Minority Member
Committee on Health, Education, Labor, and Pensions
United States Senate

The Honorable John D. Dingell
Chairman
The Honorable Joe L. Barton
Ranking Minority Member
Committee on Energy and Commerce
House of Representatives

Although children suffer from many of the same diseases as adults and are often treated with the same drugs, only about one-third of the drugs that are prescribed for children have been studied and labeled for pediatric use.[1] This has placed children taking drugs for which there have not been adequate pediatric drug studies at risk of being exposed to ineffective treatment or receiving incorrect dosing. In order to encourage the study of more drugs for pediatric use, Congress passed the Best Pharmaceuticals for Children Act (BPCA)[2] in 2002 to provide marketing incentives to drug sponsors for conducting pediatric drug studies.[3] Drug sponsors (typically drug manufacturers) may obtain 6 months of additional market exclusivity for drugs on which they have conducted pediatric studies in accordance with pertinent law and regulations.[4] This market exclusivity is known as pediatric exclusivity. When a drug has market exclusivity, it is protected from competition for a limited period, for example by prohibition on Food and Drug Administration (FDA)[5] approval of a generic copy for marketing.[6] Generally, pediatric exclusivity can only be granted to those drugs that are on-patent—that is, those that still have market exclusivity[7]—and for which FDA has issued a written request for pediatric drug studies.[8] Once a drug's patent or market exclusivity has expired, however, FDA can still request pediatric drug studies for off-patent drugs. BPCA also included provisions designed to provide for the study of both on-patent and off-patent drugs that drug sponsors have declined to study.

When FDA determines that a drug may provide health benefits to children, it may issue a written request to the drug sponsor to conduct pediatric drug studies. Under BPCA, drug sponsors of on-patent drugs must accept or decline a written request. Drug sponsors of off-patent drugs are not required to respond to a written request. However, if FDA does not receive a response within 30 days, the written request is assumed to be declined. When a drug sponsor accepts a written request for an on-patent drug and subsequently submits a study report in response, FDA generally has 90 days to complete its review of the reports to determine whether to grant pediatric exclusivity to the drug. If FDA is satisfied that the studies have been conducted and the report submitted as required, the drug in question may receive additional market exclusivity. FDA also reviews these pediatric drug study reports to see if the drug requires labeling changes. The agency refers to this review as its scientific review, which it has a goal of completing within 180 days.

BPCA provides for pediatric drug studies even if the drug sponsor declined the written request. First, if a drug sponsor declines a written request by FDA to study an on-patent drug, BPCA provides for FDA to refer the drug to the Foundation for the National Institutes of Health (FNIH), which can fund the study if funds are available.[9] When a sponsor declines a written request for an on-patent drug, the sponsor cannot receive pediatric exclusivity in response to that written request. Second, BPCA provides for the funding of the study of off-patent drugs by the Department of Health and Human Services' (HHS) National Institutes of Health (NIH).

BPCA required that we assess, among other things, the effect of provisions regarding pediatric drug studies on the study and proper labeling of drugs for pediatric use. As discussed with the committees of jurisdiction, we (1) assessed the extent to which pediatric drug studies were being conducted under BPCA for on-patent drugs, including when drug sponsors declined to conduct the studies; (2) evaluated the impact of BPCA on labeling of drugs for pediatric use and the process by which the labeling was changed; and (3) illustrated the range of diseases treated by the drugs studied under BPCA.

To assess the extent to which pediatric drug studies were being conducted under BPCA for on-patent drugs, including when drug sponsors declined to do the studies, we examined data about the drugs for which FDA issued written requests from January 2002 through December 2005. Our work focused on actions regarding these drugs prior to 2006. Specifically, we examined data on the numbers of written requests, drugs studied, written requests that were declined, and drugs granted pediatric exclusivity during this 4-year period. We reviewed data from FNIH on the funding status of on-patent drugs that drug sponsors declined to study. To evaluate the impact of BPCA on the labeling of drugs for pediatric use and the process by which labeling was changed, we reviewed summaries of the labeling changes for drugs studied from the enactment of BPCA through 2005. We reviewed the dates the labeling changes were agreed to and the reasons why some drugs did not have labeling changes. To illustrate the range of diseases treated by the drugs studied under BPCA, we identified the diseases the drugs were studied to treat, as well as the therapeutic areas addressed by the drugs. We also examined data from national surveys on the extent to which these drugs are prescribed for children. In addition, to assist with our review in general, we interviewed officials from FDA, NIH, and FNIH as well as representatives of the pharmaceutical industry and health advocates—such as the American Academy of Pediatrics, the Pharmaceutical Research and Manufacturers of America, the Generic Pharmaceutical Association, the National Organization for Rare Disorders, Public Citizen, the Elizabeth Glaser Pediatric AIDS Foundation, and the Tufts Center for the Study of Drug Development. (See app. I for a detailed description of our methodology.)

We conducted our work from September 2005 through March 2007 in accordance with generally accepted government auditing standards.

Results in Brief

Most of the on-patent drugs for which FDA requested pediatric drug studies under BPCA were being studied, but no studies resulted when the requests were declined by drug sponsors. Drug sponsors agreed to conduct studies in response to 173 of the 214 written requests for on-patent drugs (81 percent) issued by FDA from January 2002 through December 2005. Drug sponsors completed pediatric drug studies for 59 of the 173 accepted written requests—studies for the remaining 114 written requests for on-patent drugs were ongoing—and FDA made a pediatric exclusivity determination for 55 of those through December 2005. Of those 55 written requests, 52 (95 percent) resulted in FDA granting pediatric exclusivity. BPCA provides for FDA to refer the study of on-patent drugs to FNIH when drug sponsors have declined written requests. However, of the 41 written requests for on-patent drugs that drug sponsors declined to study, FDA referred 9 to FNIH, which had not funded the study of any as of December 2005.

Almost all the drugs—about 87 percent—that have been granted pediatric exclusivity under BPCA have had important labeling changes as a result of pediatric drug studies conducted under BPCA, but the process for obtaining all the necessary information, reviewing the study results, and approving these changes can be lengthy. The labeling of drugs was often changed because the pediatric drug studies revealed that children may have been exposed to ineffective drugs, ineffective dosing, overdosing, or previously unknown side effects. The review and approval process, including time for sponsors to provide needed information, took from 238 to 1,055 days when FDA required additional information to support the proposed labeling changes.

Drugs studied under BPCA were for the treatment of a wide range of diseases, including some that are common, serious, or life threatening to children. FDA identified 17 broad categories of disease that were treated by the drugs studied under BPCA. The most frequently studied drugs were those used to treat cancer, neurological and psychiatric disorders, metabolic diseases, cardiovascular disease, and viral infections. In addition, nearly half of the 10 drugs most frequently prescribed for children have been studied under BPCA.

In written comments on a draft of this report, HHS stated that the draft report provided a significant amount of data and analysis and generally explains the BPCA process, but expressed concern that it did not sufficiently acknowledge the success of BPCA or clearly describe some elements of its implementation. While assessing the overall success of BPCA was beyond the scope of this report, much of the information we present speaks to the impact BPCA has had on the studying and labeling of drugs for pediatric use. Further, we believe that we accurately presented the implementation of BPCA. We incorporated HHS's comments as appropriate.

BACKGROUND

Prior to enactment of the Food and Drug Administration Modernization Act of 1997 (FDAMA), which first established incentives for conducting pediatric drug studies in the form of additional market exclusivity, few drugs were studied for pediatric use.[10] As a result, there was a lack of information on optimal dosage, possible side effects, and the effectiveness of drugs for pediatric use. For example, while physicians typically had determined drug dosing for children based on their weight, pediatric drug studies conducted under FDAMA showed that in many cases this was not the best approach. To continue to encourage pediatric drug studies,[11] BPCA was enacted on January 4, 2002, just after the pediatric exclusivity provisions of FDAMA expired on January 1, 2002. BPCA reauthorized and enhanced the pediatric exclusivity provisions of FDAMA. Like FDAMA, BPCA allows FDA to grant drug sponsors pediatric exclusivity—6 months of additional market exclusivity—in exchange for conducting and submitting reports on pediatric drug studies. The goal of the program is to develop additional health information on the use of such drugs in pediatric populations so they can be administered safely and effectively to children. This incentive is similar to that provided by FDAMA; however, BPCA provides additional mechanisms to provide for pediatric studies of drugs that drug sponsors decline to study.

BPCA Process

The process for initiating pediatric studies under BPCA formally begins when FDA issues a written request to a drug sponsor to conduct pediatric drug studies for a particular drug. FDA may issue a written request after it has reviewed a proposed pediatric study request from a drug sponsor, in which the drug sponsor describes the pediatric drug study or studies it proposes doing in return for pediatric exclusivity. In deciding whether to approve the proposed pediatric study request and issue a written request, FDA must determine if the proposed studies will produce information that may result in health benefits for children.[12] Alternatively, FDA may determine on its own that there is a need for more research on a drug for pediatric use and issue a written request without having received a proposed pediatric study request from the drug sponsor. A written request outlines, among other things, the nature of the pediatric drug studies that the drug sponsor must conduct in order to qualify for pediatric exclusivity and a time frame by which those studies should be completed. When a drug sponsor accepts the written request and completes the pediatric drug studies, it submits reports to FDA describing the studies and the study results. BPCA specifies that FDA generally has 90 days to review the study reports to determine whether the pediatric drug studies met the conditions outlined in the written request.[13] If FDA determines that the pediatric drug studies conducted by the drug sponsor were responsive to the written request, it will grant a drug pediatric exclusivity regardless of the study findings.[14] Figure 1 illustrates the process under BPCA.

BPCA Provisions for Pediatric Drug Studies Declined by Drug Sponsors

To further the study of drugs when drug sponsors decline a written request, BPCA includes two provisions that did not exist under FDAMA. First, if a drug sponsor declines to conduct the pediatric drug studies requested by FDA for an on-patent drug, BPCA provides for FDA to refer the study of that drug to FNIH, which might then agree to fund the studies. Second, if a drug sponsor declines a request to study an off-patent drug, BPCA provides for referral of the study to

NIH for funding. FDA cannot extend pediatric exclusivity in response to written requests for any drugs for which the drug sponsor declined to conduct the requested pediatric drug studies.

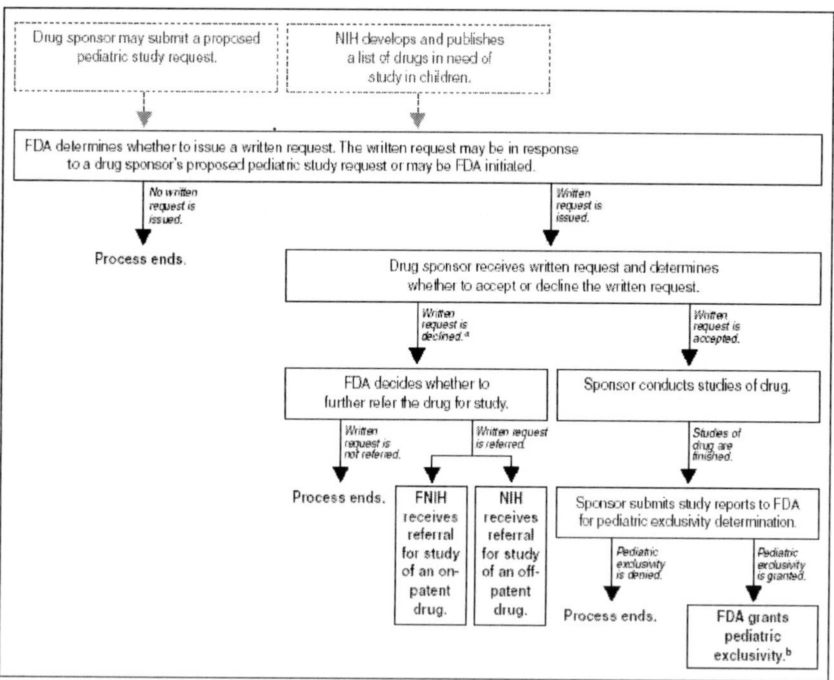

Source: GAO.

[a] If a drug sponsor of an off-patent drug does not respond to FDA's written request within 30 days, the written request is considered declined. Pediatric exclusivity is not granted to drugs where the drug sponsor declined the written request.

[b] FDA has granted pediatric exclusivity in response to written requests for on-patent drugs only. Under certain circumstances FDA could grant pediatric exclusivity in response to a written request for an off-patent drug.

Figure 1. BPCA Process

When drug sponsors decline written requests for studies of on-patent drugs, BPCA provides for FDA to refer the study of those drugs to FNIH for funding, when FDA believes that the pediatric drug studies are still warranted. FNIH, which was authorized by Congress to be established in 1990, is guided by a board of directors and began formal operations in 1996 to support the mission of NIH and advance research by linking private sector donors and partners to NIH programs. Although FNIH is a nonprofit corporation that is independent of NIH,

FNIH and NIH collaborate to fund certain projects. FNIH has raised approximately $300 million from the private sector over the past 10 years to support four general types of projects: (1) research partnerships; (2) educational programs and projects for fellows, interns, and postdoctoral students; (3) events, lectures, conferences, and communication initiatives; and (4) special projects. Included in these funds is $4.13 million that FNIH raised as of December 2005 to fund pediatric drug studies under BPCA. The majority of FNIH's funds are restricted by donors for specific projects and cannot be reallocated.[15] In recent years, appropriations of $500,000 were authorized to FNIH annually.[16]

To further the study of off-patent drugs, NIH—in consultation with FDA and other experts—develops a list of drugs, including off-patent drugs, which the agency believes are in need of study in children. NIH lists these drugs annually in the *Federal Register*. FDA may issue written requests for those drugs on the list that it determines to be most in need of study. If the drug sponsor declines or fails to respond to the written request, NIH can contract for, and fund the conduct of, the pediatric drug studies. These pediatric drug studies could then be conducted by qualified universities, hospitals, laboratories, contract research organizations, federally funded programs such as pediatric pharmacology research units, other public or private institutions or individuals. Drug sponsors generally decline written requests for off-patent drugs because the financial incentives are considerably limited. (See app. II for a description of federal efforts to encourage research on drugs for children less than 1 month of age and app. III for NIH efforts to support pediatric drug studies.)

Making Labeling Changes under BPCA for On-Patent Drugs

Pediatric drug studies often reveal new information about the safety or effectiveness of a drug, which could indicate the need for a change to its labeling. Generally, the labeling includes important information for health care providers, including proper uses of the drug, proper dosing, and possible adverse effects that could result from taking the drug. FDA may determine that the drug is not approved for use by children, which would be reflected in any labeling changes.[17]

According to FDA officials, in order to be considered for pediatric exclusivity, a drug sponsor typically submits results from pediatric drug studies in the form of a "supplemental new drug application."[18] BPCA specifies that study results, when submitted as part of a supplemental new drug application, are subject to FDA's performance goals for a scientific review, which in this case is 180 days.[19] FDA's processes for reviewing study results submitted under BPCA for consideration of labeling changes are not unique to BPCA. These are the same processes the agency would use to review any drug study results in consideration of labeling changes. FDA's action on the application can include approving the application, determining that the application is approvable (pending the submission of additional information from the sponsor), or determining that the application is not approvable. If studies demonstrate that an approved drug is not safe or effective for pediatric use, this information would be reflected in the drug's labeling.

With a determination that the application is approvable, FDA communicates to the drug sponsor that some issues need to be resolved before the application can be approved and describes what additional work is necessary to resolve the issues. This might require that drug sponsors conduct additional analyses. However, this communication would complete the scientific review cycle. When a drug sponsor resubmits the application with the additional analyses, a new scientific review cycle begins. As a result, multiple scientific review cycles might be necessary, increasing the time between initial submission of the application, which includes the pediatric study reports, and approval of a labeling change.

If, during FDA's review of the study report submitted as part of the application, the agency determines that the application is approvable and the only unresolved issue is labeling, FDA and the drug sponsor must attempt to reach agreement on labeling changes within 180 days after the application is submitted to FDA. If FDA and the drug sponsor cannot reach agreement, FDA must refer the matter to its Pediatric Advisory Committee,[20] which would convene and provide recommendations to the Commissioner on the appropriate changes to the drug's labeling. The Commissioner would then consider the committee's recommendations in making the final determination on the proper labeling.

Drug Sponsors Agreed to Study the Majority of On-Patent Drugs with Written Requests under BPCA, but No Studies Were Conducted When Drug Sponsors Declined the Written Requests

Most of the on-patent drugs for which FDA requested pediatric drug studies under BPCA were being studied, but no studies resulted when the requests were declined by drug sponsors. Of the 214 on-patent drugs for which FDA requested pediatric drug studies from January 2002 through December 2005, drug sponsors agreed to study 173 (81 percent). Of the 41 on-patent drugs that drug sponsors declined to study, FDA referred 9 to FNIH for funding and the foundation had not funded any of those studies as of December 2005.

Drug Sponsors Agreed to Conduct Pediatric Drug Studies for Most On-Patent Drugs with Written Requests Issued under BPCA

From January 2002 through December 2005, FDA issued 214 written requests for on-patent drugs to be studied under BPCA, and drug sponsors agreed to conduct pediatric drug studies for 173 (81 percent) of those.[21] The remaining 41 written requests were declined.[22] (See app. IV for details about the study of off-patent drugs under BPCA and app. V for a detailed description of the status of all written requests issued by FDA.) Drug sponsors completed pediatric drug studies for 59 of the 173 accepted written requests—studies for the remaining 114 written requests were ongoing—and FDA made a pediatric exclusivity determination for 55 of those through December 2005.[23] Of those 55 written requests, 52 (95 percent) resulted in FDA granting pediatric exclusivity.[24] Figure 2 shows the status of written requests issued under BPCA for the study of on-patent drugs, from January 2002 through December 2005. (See app. VI for a description of the complexity of pediatric drug studies conducted under BPCA.)

FNIH Had Not Funded the Study of Any On-Patent Drugs in Children

Under BPCA, when a written request to study an on-patent drug is declined, the study of the drug may be referred to FNIH. However, FNIH is limited in its ability to fund drug studies by its available funds. Through December 2005, drug sponsors declined written requests issued under BPCA for 41 on-patent drugs. FDA referred 9 of these 41 written requests (22 percent) to FNIH for funding.[25] FNIH had not funded the study of any of these drugs.[26] NIH has estimated that the cost of studying the drugs that were referred to FNIH for study would exceed $43 million (see table 1). FNIH has been raising funds for the study of drugs referred under BCPA at a rate of approximately $1 million per year.

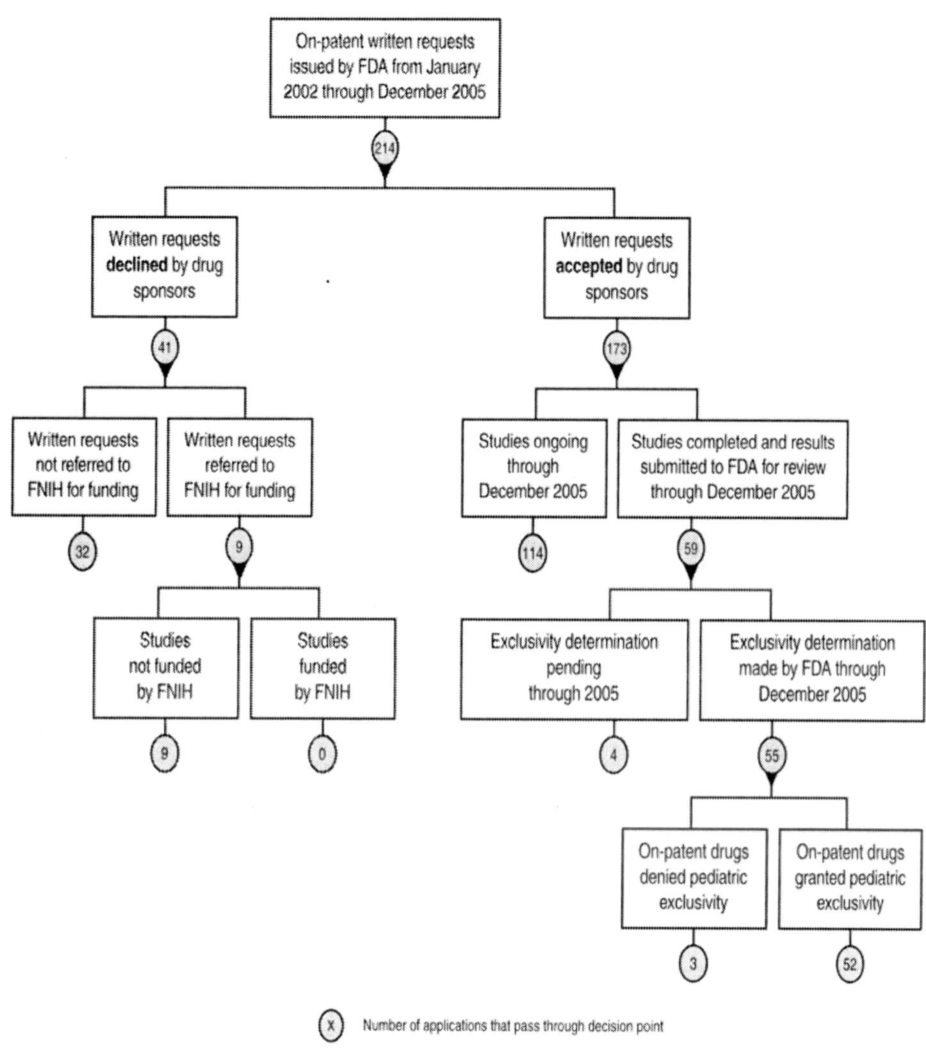

Source: GAO.

Note: Written requests issued from January 2002 through December 2005 include new written requests issued under BPCA combined with written requests originally issued under FDAMA but reissued under BPCA.

Figure 2. Status of Written Requests Issued under BPCA for the Study of On-Patent Drugs, from January 2002 through December 2005

Table 1. Estimated Costs of Funding the Study of On-Patent Drugs Referred to FNIH under BPCA

On-patent drug	Disease or condition to be studied	Estimated cost
Baclofen	Spasticity in children with cerebral palsy	$7.8 million
Bupropion	Depression	$7.4 million
Dexrazoxane	Used to block the cardiac effects of the anticancer drug adriamycin	Not provided[a]
Eletriptan	Migraine headaches	Not provided[a]
Hydroxyurea[b]	Sickle cell disease	$8 million to $10 million[c]
Metoclopramide	Gastroesophageal reflux disease	Not provided[a]
Morphine	Analgesia	$8.7 million
Sevelamer	Renal failure	$2.7 million
Zonisamide	Refractory partial seizures	$8.4 million
Total		**$43 million to $45 million[d]**

Source: NIH.

[a] Cost estimates have not been provided by NIH.

[b] Hydroxyurea is available in on-patent and generic (or off-patent) formulations. According to NIH officials, after the written request was referred to FNIH for funding, NIH determined that a study funded by its National Heart, Lung, and Blood Institute would provide much of the needed information for appropriate pediatric use. In 2005, NIH's National Institute of Child Health and Human Development agreed to cofund the study.

[c] A formal cost estimate has not been made by NIH, but an initial estimate ranged from $8 million to $10 million.

[d] Total estimated cost is for the six drugs for which an estimated cost is available.

Most Drugs Granted Pediatric Exclusivity under BPCA Had Labeling Changes, but the Process for Making Changes Was Sometimes Lengthy

Most drugs—about 87 percent—that have been granted pediatric exclusivity under BPCA have had labeling changes as a result of the pediatric drug studies conducted under BPCA. Pediatric drug studies conducted under BPCA showed that children may have been exposed to ineffective drugs, ineffective dosing, overdosing, or side effects that were previously unknown. However, the process for reviewing study results and completing labeling changes was sometimes lengthy, particularly when FDA required additional information to support the changes.

Most Drugs Granted Pediatric Exclusivity Had Labeling Changes

Of the 52 drugs studied and granted pediatric exclusivity under BPCA from January 2002 through December 2005, 45 (about 87 percent) had labeling changes as a result of the pediatric drug studies. FDA officials told us that labeling changes were not made for the remaining 7 (about 13 percent) drugs granted pediatric exclusivity, generally because data provided by the pediatric drug studies did not support labeling changes. In addition, 3 other drugs had labeling changes prior to FDA making a decision on granting pediatric exclusivity.[27] FDA officials said these labeling changes were made prior to determining whether pediatric exclusivity should be granted because the pediatric drug studies provided important safety information that should be reflected in the labeling without waiting until the full study results were submitted or pediatric exclusivity was determined.

Labeling Changes for Drugs Studied under BPCA Had Important Implications for Pediatric Use

Pediatric drug studies conducted under BPCA have shown that the way that some drugs were being administered to children potentially exposed them to an ineffective therapy, ineffective dosing, overdosing, or previously unknown side effects—including some that affect growth and development. The labeling for these drugs was changed to reflect these study results. Table 2 shows some of these drugs and illustrates these types of labeling changes. FDA officials said that the agency has been working to increase the amount of information included in drug labeling, particularly when pediatric drug studies indicate that an approved drug may not be safe or effective for pediatric use.

Table 2. Examples of Labeling Changes

Potential risks or hazards	Drug name	Disease or condition treated	Summary of new information contained in drug labeling
Unnecessary exposure to ineffective therapies	Sumatriptan	Migraines	Five studies did not establish safety and effectiveness, and postmarketing experience showed children were having serious adverse effects, such as stroke and vision loss. The product is not recommended for children under 18 years old.
	Tolterodine	Overactive bladder and urge incontinence	The drug was not shown to be effective for children and appeared to show a possible increase in aggressive, hyperactive, and abnormal behavior.
	Irinotecan	Tumors	Children had more rapid disease progression and died more quickly. The labeling states that the drug should not be used to treat children with a particular kind of tumor.
Ineffective dosing	Oxcarbazepine	Partial seizures	Dose for children aged 2 to 4 and weighing less than 44 po-unds is twice the dose per bo-dy weight compared to adults.
	Methylphenidate	Attention-deficit hyperactivity disorder	Children aged 13 to 17 elimi-nated the drug from their bod-ies faster than the comparison age group. Therefore the dos-ing regimen may be increased to prevent ineffective dosing.

Table 2. (Continued)

Potential risks or hazards	Drug name	Disease or condition treated	Summary of new information contained in drug labeling
Overdosing	Leflunomide	Juvenile rheumatoid arthritis	Children weighing less than 88 pounds require a lower-than-expected dose. Over-dosing leflunomide, which has significant toxicity, could make the drug's risks to chil-dren outweigh its benefits.
Previously unlabeled side effects, including effect on growth and development	Venlafaxine	Depression; generalized anxiety disorder	This drug is associated with an increased risk of suicidal thinking and behavior.
	Ciprofloxacin	Complicated urinary tract infection or kidney infection	This drug is associated with increased adverse effects to joints or surrounding tissues for children.
	Fentanyl	Chronic pain	This drug should be used only by children who are 2 years of age or older and are opioid-tolerant. Use by others can lead to life-threatening respi-ratory depression and death.
	Budesonide	Asthma	Budesonide can cause growth suppression.

Source: GAO analysis of FDA data.

Other drugs have had labeling changes indicating that the drug may be used safely and effectively by children in certain dosages or forms. Typically, this resulted in the drug labeling being changed to indicate that the drug was approved for use by children younger than those for whom it had previously been approved. In other cases, the changes reflected a new formulation of a drug, such as a syrup that was developed for pediatric use, or new directions for preparing the drug for pediatric use were identified during the pediatric drug studies conducted under BPCA.[28] (See table 3 for examples of drugs with this new type of information.)

Table 3. Examples of Drugs Approved for Use by Younger Children or for Which New Formulations Are Available

Uses and formulations	Drug	Disease or condition treated or prevented	Summary of new information
New age groups	Moxifloxacin Ophthalmic	Bacterial conjunctivitis	Found to be safe and effective for children over 1 year old.
	Ondansetron	Nausea and vomiting after chemotherapy	Established dosing for surgical patients down to 1 month from 2 years of age; established dosing for cancer patients down to 6 months from 4 years of age.
New formulations or preparations	Benazepril	Hypertension	Labeled with directions for how to prepare a suspension for administering the drug to children.
	Desloratadine	Seasonal and perennial allergic rhinitis and hives	Newly available in a syrup, labeled specifically for children.

Source: GAO analysis.

The Process for Reviewing Study Results and Approving Labeling Changes Was Sometimes Lengthy, Particularly When FDA Required Additional Information from Drug Sponsors

Although FDA generally completed its first scientific review of study results submitted as a supplemental new drug application—including consideration of labeling changes—within its 180-day goal, the process for completing the review, including obtaining sufficient information to support and approve labeling changes, sometimes took longer. For the 45 drugs granted pediatric exclusivity that had labeling changes, it took an average of almost 9 months after study results were first submitted to FDA for the sponsor to submit and the agency to review all of the information it required and agree with the drug sponsor to approve the labeling changes.[29] For 13 drugs (about 29 percent), FDA completed this scientific review process and FDA approved labeling changes within 180 days. It took from 181 to 187 days to complete the scientific review process and to approve labeling changes for 14 drugs (about 31 percent). For the remaining 18 drugs (about 40 percent), it took from 238 to 1,055 days for FDA to complete the scientific review process and approve labeling changes. For 7 of those drugs, it took more than a year to complete the scientific review process and approve labeling changes.

To determine whether and how drug labeling should be changed, FDA conducts a scientific review of the study results that are submitted to the agency by the drug sponsor. Included with the study results is the drug sponsor's proposal for how the labeling should be changed. FDA can either accept the proposed wording or propose alternative wording. For some drugs, however, the process does not end with FDA's first scientific review. While the first scientific reviews were generally completed within 180 days, for the 18 drugs that took 238 days or more, FDA determined that it needed additional information from the drug sponsors in order to be able to approve the applications. This often required that the drug sponsors conduct additional analyses or pediatric drug studies. FDA officials said they could not approve any changes to drug labeling until the drug sponsors provided this information. When FDA completed its review of the information that was originally submitted and requested additional information from the drug sponsors, the initial 180-day scientific review ended. A new 180-day scientific review began when the drug sponsors submitted the additional information to FDA. Drug sponsors sometimes took as long as 1 year to gather the additional necessary data and respond to FDA's requests. This time did not count against FDA's 180-day goal to complete its scientific review and approve labeling changes because a new 180-day scientific review begins after the required information is submitted. However, we counted the total number of days between submission of study reports and approval of labeling changes. FDA considers itself in conformance with its review goals even though the entire process may take longer than 180 days.

BPCA provides a dispute resolution process to be used if FDA and the drug sponsor cannot reach agreement on labeling changes within 180 days of when FDA received the application and the only issue holding up FDA approval is the wording of the drug labeling. However, FDA officials said they have never used this process because labeling has never been the only unresolved issue for those applications whose review period exceeded 180 days. Agency officials told us that the possibility of referral to the Pediatric Advisory Committee facilitates its negotiations with drug sponsors on labeling changes because it is something that drug sponsors want to avoid. Reminding the drug sponsors that such a process exists has motivated drug sponsors to complete labeling change negotiations by reaching agreement with FDA. (See app. VII for a discussion of strengths of BPCA identified by FDA and NIH, as well as suggestions for ways to improve BPCA.)

Drugs Studied under BPCA Address a Wide Range of Diseases, Including Some That Are Common, Serious, or Life Threatening to Children

Drugs were studied under BPCA for their safety and effectiveness in treating children for a wide range of diseases, including some that are common, serious, or life threatening. We found that the drugs studied under BPCA represented more than 17 broad categories of disease. The category that had the most drugs studied under BPCA was cancer, with 28 drugs. In addition, there were 26 drugs studied for neurological and psychiatric disorders, 19 for endocrine and metabolic disorders, 18 related to cardiovascular disease—including drugs related to hypertension, and 17 related to viral infections. Written requests for some types of drugs were more frequently declined by the drug sponsor than others. For example, 36 percent of written requests for pulmonary drugs and 41 percent of written requests for drugs that treat nonviral infection were declined. In contrast, 19 percent of written requests were declined overall.

Some of the drugs studied under BPCA were for the treatment of diseases that are common, including those for the treatment of asthma and allergies. Analysis of two national databases shows that about half of the 10 most frequently prescribed drugs for children were studied under BPCA. Based on a survey of prescriptions written by physicians in 2004, 4 of the 10 drugs most frequently prescribed for children were studied under BPCA.[30] A survey of families and their medical providers in 2003 found that 5 of the 10 drugs most frequently prescribed for children were studied under BPCA.[31] In addition, several of the drugs studied under BPCA were for the treatment of diseases that are serious or life threatening to children, such as hypertension, cancer, HIV, and influenza. Table 4 provides information on some of the drugs studied for pediatric use and what is known about the diseases that are relevant to children.

Some of the drugs were studied under BPCA to treat complicating conditions in children who had other diseases, while others treated rare diseases. For example a drug was studied for the treatment of painful bladder spasms in children who have spina bifida. Other drugs were studied to treat overactive bladder symptoms in children with spina bifida and cerebral palsy, to treat children who require chronic pain management because of severe illnesses such as cancer, and to treat partial seizures and epilepsy in children who require more than one drug to control seizures. About 12 percent of the 52 drugs that were granted pediatric exclusivity under BPCA were studied for the treatment of rare diseases, including certain types of leukemia, juvenile rheumatoid arthritis, and narcolepsy.

Table 4. Examples of Diseases to Be Treated by Drugs Studied under BPCA

Specific disease treated by drug	Information about the disease
Allergies	Allergies affect up to 40 percent of, or about 29 million, children in the United States.
Asthma	Asthma affects 6.2 million or 9 percent of children in the United States. Further, asthma is the most common chronic illness among children.
Cancer	Cancer is the leading cause of death by disease for children aged 1 to 14 in the United States.
HIV	About 20 percent of HIV-infected children worldwide develop serious disease before they turn 1, and most of those die before age 4. Through the end of 2002, 9,300 children under age 13 in the United States were living with HIV.
Hypertension	An estimated 3.25 million (4.5 percent) children in the United States have high blood pressure. Untreated, high blood pressure can lead to damage to the heart, brain, kidneys, and eyes.
Influenza	Population-based studies show that 15 to 42 percent of preschool and school-aged children contract the flu. Influenza can have serious complications for children, including pneumonia and dehydration, and can lead to death. In the 2003-2004 flu season, more United States children died from the flu than chicken pox, whooping cough, and measles combined, and nearly two-thirds were under the age of 5.

Source: GAO analysis.

Note: Based on data published from 2000 through 2006.

AGENCY COMMENTS AND OUR EVALUATION

HHS provided written comments on a draft of this report, which we have reprinted in appendix VIII. HHS stated that the draft report provided a significant amount of data and analysis and generally explains the BPCA process. HHS also made four general comments. First, HHS commented that the report does not sufficiently acknowledge the success of BPCA. HHS noted that BPCA provides additional incentives for the study of on-patent drugs, a process for the study of off-patent drugs, a safety review of all drugs granted pediatric exclusivity, and the public dissemination of information from pediatric studies conducted. HHS concluded that BPCA has generated more clinical information for the pediatric population than any other legislative or regulatory effort to date. Second, HHS commented that the report confuses FDA's process for reviewing reports of drug studies conducted under BPCA with time frames for the labeling dispute resolution process outlined in BPCA. HHS suggested that we did not sufficiently acknowledge that some of the time it takes for FDA to approve labeling changes includes time spent by sponsors collecting and submitting additional information. Third, in commenting on our finding that few written requests included neonates, HHS pointed out that written requests for 9 drugs required the inclusion of "newborns" and written requests for 13 drugs required the inclusion of infants (children under 4 months of age). Fourth, HHS commented that we failed to mention that exclusivity attaches to patents as well as existing market exclusivity.

We believe that the draft report sent to HHS for comment accurately and adequately addressed each of the four issues upon which HHS commented. An explicit discussion of the overall success of BPCA was outside the scope of this report, as directed by the BPCA mandate and as discussed with the committees of jurisdiction. Nevertheless, the draft report extensively discussed HHS accomplishments such as the number of studies conducted, the number and importance of labeling changes that FDA approved, and the wide range of diseases, including some that are common, serious, or life threatening to children, for which drugs were studied.

In drafting our report we believe we clearly distinguished between FDA's goals for completing its review and approval of drug applications and the time frames mandated for using the labeling dispute resolution process as outlined in BPCA. In finding that the process for approving labeling changes is lengthy, we clearly stated that the process included time spent during FDA's initial review as well as time drug sponsors took to respond to FDA's requests for additional information, which was as long as 1 year. We also acknowledged that FDA completed its initial review of applications within its 180-day goal. We stated in the draft that FDA has never used the dispute resolution process because labeling has never been the only issue preventing FDA's approval of a label for more than 180 days. Nevertheless, we have included additional language in this report to further clarify the distinction between FDA's review process for pediatric applications and labeling dispute resolution.

Our draft clearly stated that while written requests issued under BPCA required the inclusion of neonates, the majority of those on-patent written requests—32 of 36—had been first issued under FDAMA. It is therefore not appropriate to attribute the inclusion of neonates in these written requests to BPCA. Further, we included in our count of written requests requiring the inclusion of neonates the 9 written requests that HHS referred to in its comments as requiring the inclusion of newborns. We did not specifically include in our counts the other 13 written requests mentioned in HHS's comments. According to data provided by FDA, 1 of these written requests was not issued under BPCA, and 2 others were counted among the 9 mentioned above. The remaining 10 written requests were not specifically included in our counts, because the written requests were first issued prior to BPCA and do not specifically require the inclusion of neonates. The written requests to which HHS referred in its comments required the inclusion of very young children, age 0-4 months. Our draft report had indicated that written requests requiring the inclusion of young children might produce data about neonates.

Our draft report included language that indicated the conditions under which pediatric exclusivity applies. We added language to the report to further clarify the conditions under which pediatric exclusivity can be granted.

HHS provided technical comments which we incorporated as appropriate. HHS also stated that many of the oral comments provided by FDA were not reflected in the draft report sent to HHS for formal comment. Some of FDA's suggested revisions and comments were outside the scope of the report and in some instances we chose to use alternative wording to that suggested by FDA for readability and consistency. As we did with HHS's general and technical comments on this report, we previously incorporated FDA's oral comments as appropriate.

We are sending copies of this report to the Secretary of Health and Human Services, appropriate congressional committees, and other interested parties. We will also make copies available to others upon request. In addition, the report will be available at no charge on GAO's Web site at http://www.gao.gov . If you have any questions about this report, please contact me at (202) 512-7119 or crossem@gao.gov . Contact points for our Offices of Congressional Relations and

Public Affairs may be found on the last page of this report. GAO staff who made major contributions to this report are listed in appendix IX.

Marcia Crosse
Director, Health Care

APPENDIX I: SCOPE AND METHODOLOGY

In this report, we (1) assessed the extent to which pediatric drug studies were being conducted for on-patent drugs under the Best Pharmaceuticals for Children Act (BPCA), including when drug sponsors declined to conduct the studies; (2) evaluated the impact of BPCA on labeling of drugs for pediatric use and the process by which the labeling was changed; and (3) illustrated the range of diseases treated by the drugs studied under BPCA.

Our review focused primarily on those on-patent drugs for which written requests were issued or reissued by the Department of Health and Human Services' (HHS) Food and Drug Administration (FDA) from January 2002, when BPCA was enacted, through December 2005. Actions taken on these drugs after December 2005 (such as a determination of pediatric exclusivity or a labeling change) were not included in our review. In addition, we reviewed some summary data available about the number of written requests issued under the Food and Drug Administration Modernization Act of 1997 (FDAMA) from January 1998 through December 2001. We also reviewed pertinent laws, regulations, and legislative histories.

To assess the extent to which pediatric drug studies were being conducted for on-patent drugs under BPCA, including when the drug sponsors declined to conduct the studies, we identified written requests issued for on-patent drugs from January 2002 through December 2005, and determined which of those were declined by drug sponsors. We also reviewed data provided by FDA on the nature of the pediatric drug studies that were conducted in response to the written requests issued under BPCA. We also examined notices published in the *Federal Register*, identifying the drugs designated by HHS's National Institutes of Health (NIH) as most in need of study in children. We reviewed data provided to us by the Foundation for the National Institutes of Health (FNIH)—a nonprofit corporation independent of NIH—about funding for pediatric drug studies of on-patent drugs. We interviewed officials from FDA, NIH, and FNIH to understand the processes by which pediatric drug studies are prioritized by the agencies, written requests are issued, drug sponsors respond to written requests, study results are submitted to FDA, and pediatric exclusivity determinations are made. We also reviewed background material describing the role of FNIH in supporting research on children and the funding available for such research.

To evaluate the impact of BPCA on the labeling of drugs for pediatric use and the process by which the labeling was changed, we reviewed data provided to us by FDA summarizing the changes made from January 2002 through December 2005 for drugs studied under BPCA. We also used the dates that the changes were approved in order to calculate how long it took for FDA to approve labeling changes. We interviewed officials from FDA about the process by which FDA approves labeling changes as well as the reasons why some drugs did not have labeling changes.

To illustrate the range of diseases treated by the drugs studied under BPCA, we reviewed data provided by FDA about the disease each drug was proposed to treat. We also examined data from the Medical Expenditure Panel Survey—administered by the Agency for Healthcare Research and Quality—and the National Ambulatory Medical Care Survey—administered by the National Center for Health Statistics—to assess the extent to which the drugs studied under BPCA were prescribed to children.

To obtain other information that is provided in appendixes to this report, we collected and analyzed a variety of data from FDA, NIH, and FNIH about written requests and pediatric studies for both on- and off-patent drugs. To obtain a broad perspective on the many issues addressed in our report, we also interviewed representatives of the pharmaceutical industry and health advocates—such as representatives of the American Academy of Pediatrics, the Pharmaceutical Research and Manufacturers of America, the Generic Pharmaceutical Association, the National Organization of Rare Disorders, Public Citizen, the Elizabeth Glaser Pediatric AIDS Foundation, and the Tufts Center for the Study of Drug Development.

We evaluated the data used in this report and determined that they were sufficiently reliable for our purposes. We conducted our work from September 2005 through March 2007 in accordance with generally accepted government auditing standards.

APPENDIX II: FDA AND NIH EFFORTS TO ENCOURAGE THE STUDY OF DRUGS IN NEONATES SINCE PASSAGE OF BPCA

FDA and NIH have engaged in efforts to increase the inclusion of neonates—children under the age of 1 month—in pediatric drug studies. As part of its encouragement of pediatric studies in general, BPCA identified neonates as a specific group to be included in studies, as appropriate. An examination of the written requests revealed that only 4 of 36 written requests for on-patent drugs first issued under BPCA required the inclusion of neonates. Further, no written requests for on-patent drugs and only two written requests for off-patent drugs have required the inclusion of neonates since FDA and NIH held a workshop that began their major initiative in this regard in 2004.

NIH Workshops

In 2003, NIH conducted three workshops focused on increasing the inclusion of neonates in pediatric drug studies and discussing diseases that affect neonates. In September 2003, NIH staff met to discuss drug studies in neonatology and pediatrics with special emphasis placed on ways to better apply current knowledge in future pediatric drug studies. Two months later, NIH met with a group of experts to discuss the use of the drug dobutamine—used to treat low blood pressure—in neonates. NIH ended 2003 with a 1-day seminar designed to address parental attitudes toward neonatal clinical trials.

NIH Initiatives

FDA and NIH have collaborated to develop the Newborn Drug Development Initiative (NDDI), a multiphase program intended to identify gaps in knowledge concerning neonatal pharmacology and pediatric drug study design and to explore novel designs for studies of drugs for use by neonates. The NDDI is intended to consist of a series of meetings that will help frame state-of-the-art approaches and research needs. After forming various discussion groups in February 2003, the agencies held a workshop in March 2004 to help frame issues and challenges associated with designing and conducting drug studies with neonates. The workshop addressed ethical issues and drug prioritization in four specialty areas: pain control, pulmonology (the study of conditions affecting the lungs and breathing), cardiology (the study of conditions affecting the heart), and neurology (the study of disorders of the brain and central nervous system). For example, participants in the pain control group reviewed data demonstrating that neonates who undergo multiple painful procedures and receive medication to treat pain may differ in their development of pain receptors compared to those who do not undergo such procedures and treatment. FDA officials said that FDA would apply the findings from the NDDI workshop to written requests for pediatric drug studies in the four specialty areas.

NIH officials said that the Pediatric Formulations Initiative is a related effort. They said that both initiatives are long-standing activities that engage in various efforts to enhance information dissemination to improve all pediatric drug studies. According to NIH officials, these initiatives have resulted in numerous publications.

Pediatric Drug Studies Requiring the Study of Neonates

FDA and NIH efforts to increase the inclusion of neonates in pediatric drug studies conducted under BPCA have been limited. Through 2005, 9 of 16 (56 percent) written requests for off-patent drugs required the inclusion of neonates in the pediatric drug studies. NIH is currently funding pediatric drug studies for four of these written requests. Similarly, 36 of 214 (17 percent) written requests for the study of on-patent drugs issued from January 2002 through December 2005 included a requirement to study neonates, but only 4 of those 36 (11 percent) were first issued under BPCA. The remaining 32 (89 percent) written requests were originally issued under FDAMA, which did not place an emphasis on the inclusion of neonates in pediatric drug studies. Further, all of the written requests requiring the inclusion of neonates were issued in 2003, prior to the NDDI. Further, only two of the written requests for off-patent drugs were issued after the NDDI, and studies for neither of those have been funded. According to information provided by FDA, no written requests for on-patent drugs issued from January 2004 through December 2005 required the inclusion of neonates. FDA officials indicated, however, that they receive information about neonates in response to written requests that do not specifically target them. According to these officials, many written requests require that children from birth through 2 years of age be studied. These pediatric drug studies therefore may include neonates. In addition, inclusion of neonates in some studies may not be appropriate for medical or ethical reasons.

Appendix III: NIH Efforts to Support Pediatric Drug Studies

BPCA was designed in part to increase pediatric drug studies through federal efforts. NIH has engaged in several efforts to support pediatric drug studies since the passage of BPCA.

NIH Funding

While NIH plays an important role in providing funding for research for children, the amount provided by NIH to support such activities has not increased significantly under BPCA. Since the enactment of BPCA, NIH funding for children's research has increased from $3.1 billion in fiscal year 2003 to $3.2 billion in fiscal year 2005. These figures represent about 11 percent of NIH's total budget each year from 2003 through 2005. The research funds for children were distributed by most of NIH's 28 institutes, centers, and offices.[32] For example, in 2005, 24 of these institutes, centers, and offices funded research on children. One institute, the National Institute of Child Health and Human Development, was responsible for about 26 percent of funding for pediatric research—the largest proportion of NIH's research funding for children. This institute organizes study design teams with FDA and other relevant NIH institutes, conducts contracting activities, and modifies drug labeling for specific ages and diseases.

Pediatric Pharmacology Research Units

The number of pediatric pharmacology research units—initiated by NIH—devoted to studies for children has remained the same under BPCA.[33] NIH provides about $500,000 annually to each of these research units to provide the infrastructure for independent investigators to initiate and collaborate on studies and clinical trials with private industry and NIH. The number of such research units grew from 7 in 1994 to 13 in 1999 to support the infrastructure for collaborative efforts of pharmacologists to conduct clinical trials that include children. While the number has not changed since the passage of BPCA in 2002, NIH officials said that staff from these units often move on to hospitals throughout the country and enhance the pediatric research capacity nationwide. In addition, they said that an overall increase in pediatric research capacity nationwide in recent years has made it possible to conduct pediatric clinical trials at a number of other sites. They said that, on average, these pediatric pharmacology research units conduct more than 50 pediatric drug studies annually. Of these, as many as 20 pediatric drug studies are funded by drug sponsors. NIH officials told us that of the seven off-patent drugs being studied under BPCA with NIH funding through 2005, two were being conducted by these research units. NIH officials said that since on-patent written requests are not published, the full contribution of the research units under BPCA cannot be ascertained.

Table 5. NIH-Sponsored Activities, Through 2005, Related to Children in Clinical Trials

Year(s)	Activity focus
2002, 2003, 2004, 2005	Pediatric experts offered advice to NIH concerning drugs that should be studied for use by children, leading to the published list of off-patent drugs in the *Federal Register*.
2003	Discussed ways to improve access to information on the frequency of medication use by children and improve the list development process surrounding the measurement of this frequency.
2003	Discussed ways to use current knowledge to better inform future studies of drugs in children.
2003	Discussed the use of two drugs, dobutamine and dopamine, in neonates.
2003	Discussed parent attitudes toward studies of neonates and other issues related to the consent for studies in children.
2004	Explored diverse models useful in understanding efficacy and toxicity of drugs across the course of development.
2005	Discussed the development of treatment strategies and recommendations for drugs to be studied in managing pediatric hypertension.
2005	Reviewed and analyzed databases used to describe the frequency of health conditions leading families to seek care for their children in different outpatient health care delivery settings, such as pediatric clinics and offices, and inpatient hospital settings. Those conditions leading to death were also part of the review.
2005	Reviewed and analyzed databases available to describe the frequency of use of medications by children in outpatient delivery settings.
2005	Discussed challenges from lack of appropriate pediatric formulations and improvements of pediatric therapeutics.

Source: NIH.

Meetings and Forums

NIH has sponsored a number of forums designed to increase the number of children included in drug studies. As shown in table 5, these forums generated advice and suggestions for NIH concerning drug testing from health experts, process improvements on drug studies and medication use with the pediatric community, and explanations of models and data related to research for children.

NIH has also conducted meetings and entered numerous intra-agency and FDA agreements to strengthen its relationship with FDA and establish a firm commitment to study medical issues relevant to children. For example, NIH conducted a series of internal meetings in fiscal year 2004 to identify ongoing pediatric drug studies by the National Institute of Mental Health. As an outcome of these meetings, NIH identified and utilized data sets related to the study of lithium as it is used for the treatment of bipolar disorder in children. NIH will use this information to enhance its current understanding of the drug's therapeutic benefit.

APPENDIX IV: STUDIES OF OFF-PATENT DRUGS UNDER BPCA

In addition to providing a mechanism to study on-patent drugs, BPCA also contains provisions for the study of off-patent drugs. FDA initiates its process by issuing a written request to the drug sponsor to study an off-patent drug. If the sponsor declines to study the drug, FDA can refer the study of the drug to NIH for funding. NIH initiates the BPCA process for off-patent drugs by prioritizing the list of drugs that need to be studied.

Written Requests for Studies of Off-Patent Drugs under BPCA

BPCA includes a provision that provides for the funding of the study of off-patent drugs by NIH. BPCA requires that NIH—in consultation with FDA and other experts—publish an annual list of drugs for which additional studies are needed to assess their safety and effectiveness in children.[34] FDA can then issue a written request for pediatric studies of the off-patent drugs on the list. If the written request is declined by the drug sponsor, NIH can fund the studies.

Few off-patent drugs identified by NIH as in need of study for pediatric use have been studied. From 2003 through 2006, NIH has listed off-patent drugs that were recommended for study by experts in pediatric research and clinical practice.[35] By 2005, NIH had identified 40 off-patent drugs that it believed should be studied for pediatric use.[36] Through 2005, FDA issued written requests for 16 of these drugs.[37] All but one of these written requests were declined by drug sponsors. NIH funded pediatric drug studies for 7 of the remaining 15 written requests declined by drug sponsors through December 2005.

NIH provided several reasons why it has not pursued the study of some off-patent drugs that drug sponsors declined to study. Concerns about the incidence of the diseases that the drugs were developed to treat, the feasibility of study design, drug safety, and changes in the drugs' patent status have caused the agency to reconsider the merit of studying some of the drugs it identified as important for study in children.[38] For example, in one case NIH issued a request for proposals to study a drug but received no response. In other cases, NIH is awaiting consultation with pediatric experts to determine the potential for study.

Further, NIH has not received appropriations specifically for funding pediatric drug studies under BPCA. Rather, according to agency officials, NIH uses lump sum appropriations made to various institutes to fund pediatric drug studies under BPCA. In fiscal year 2005, NIH spent approximately $25 million for these pediatric drug studies.

Funding for Studies of Off-Patent Drugs under BPCA

NIH anticipates spending an estimated $52.5 million for pediatric drug studies following seven written requests to drug sponsors issued by FDA from January 2002 through December 2005.[39] These pediatric drug studies were designed to take from 3 to 4 years and will be completed in 2007 at the earliest. Where possible, NIH identifies another government agency or institute within NIH that might be able to meet the requirements of the written requests and conduct the pediatric drug studies. In cases where a government agency will conduct the pediatric drug studies, NIH institutes enter into intra- or interagency agreements for the studies. If those efforts fail, the agency develops and publishes requests for proposals for others to conduct the pediatric studies.

Table 6. Anticipated NIH Spending for Off-Patent Drug Studies Committed to through 2005

Drug	Total cost[a]	Disease or condition	Funded agency or organization	Anticipated completion
Studies for drugs with a written request				
Dactinomycin[b]	$1,800,000[c]	Cancer	Children's Oncology Group through the National Cancer Institute	2007
Hydroxyurea	$7,000,000[c]	Sickle cell	National Heart Lung and Blood Institute	2008
Lithium	$17,400,000[c]	Mania in bipolar disorder	Case Western University	2008
Lorazepam (two diseases/conditions)	$15,100,000[d]	Status epilepticus (seizures)	National Institutes of Health	2008
		Sedation	National Institutes of Health	2008
Sodium nitroprusside	$9,400,000[c]	Control of blood pressure	Stanford University and Duke University	2007
Vincristine[b]	$1,800,000[c]	Malignancies	Children's Oncology Group through the National Cancer Institute	2007
Subtotal	**$52,500,000**			
Studies initiated prior to a written request[e]				
Daunomycin (Daunorubicin)	$1,400,000[c]	Cancer	Children's Oncology Group through the National Cancer Institute	2008
Ketamine	$1,000,000[d]	Sedation	FDA's National Center for Toxicological Research	2008
Methotrexate	$8,900,000[d]	Cancer	Children's Oncology Group through the National Cancer Institute	2009
Methylphenidate	$4,700,000[f]	Attention deficit hyperactivity disorder	National Institute of Environmental Health Sciences	2007
Subtotal	**$16,000,000**			
Total	**$68,500,000**			

Source: GAO analysis of NIH data.

[a] Total costs proposed for most studies are estimates and may vary over time because of modifications of initial projects, rounded to the nearest $100,000.

[b] Dactinomycin and Vincristine are commonly used together and the cost to study both is $3,600,000.

[c] Studies to be completed over 3 years.

[d] Studies to be completed over 4 years.

[e] No written request was issued by FDA for the specific studies prior to being funded by NIH. Ketamine is listed in the *Federal Register* as a drug in need of study in children (69 *Fed. Reg.* 7243-44, Feb. 13, 2004). Because of data demonstrating that ketamine enhances cell death in the brain in animals, it is not possible to design an ethical study using children. Ketamine has since been listed in the *Federal Register* as having preclinical toxicology studies under way, with clinical studies awaiting their completion (71 *Fed. Reg.* 23931-36, Apr. 25, 2006). Methylphenidate was selected, though it is not included on the list published in the *Federal Register*, because of a potentially serious public health concern that arose unexpectedly. HHS officials reported that studies on ketamine and methylphenidate are not the type that typically would be requested under BPCA, nor was a written request issued for these specific studies. Daunomycin and methotrexate were selected prior to being listed in the *Federal Register* because the National Cancer Institute had access to the appropriate children for study and was developing studies that would produce data for both drugs.

[f] Studies to be completed over 2 years.

NIH anticipates spending approximately $16.0 million for the funding of pediatric drug studies of four additional off-patent drugs for which FDA did not issue written requests—and therefore are not covered by the requirements of BPCA—but three of these drugs have since been listed by NIH in the *Federal Register* as needing study in children.[40] (See table 6.)

The drugs whose study NIH is funding without written requests were selected because of special circumstances that raised their priority for funding. NIH funded the study of daunomycin and methotrexate—both cancer drugs—before placing them on its 2006 list of drugs for study in children. NIH officials told us that the Children's Oncology Group of the National Cancer Institute was already working with an appropriate group of patients and was at a critical stage in developing the pediatric drug studies that would produce data for both drugs, so pediatric drug studies were funded before the drugs were placed on the priority list. NIH officials also told us that ketamine is administered to more than 30,000 children for sedation each year. Studies done in animals, however, have suggested that the drug may lead to cell death in the brain. As a result, the drug cannot be ethically tested in children. NIH is therefore collaborating with FDA to conduct studies in nonhuman primates. NIH officials report that methylphenidate is used by an estimated 2.5 million school-aged children to treat attention deficit hyperactivity disorder. However, a recent study suggested some potential genetic toxicity of the drug. Because of these findings, the drug was targeted as a priority and NIH was able to fund some of the planned studies related to this drug.

Appendix V: Status of Pediatric Drug Studies Requested by FDA

From January 2002 through December 2005, FDA issued 214 written requests for the study of on-patent drugs. The agency also issued 16 written requests for the study of off-patent drugs. Fewer written requests were issued and more were declined by drug sponsors under BPCA than under FDAMA.

Written Requests Issued under BPCA Compared to FDAMA

From January 2002, when BPCA was enacted, through December 2005, FDA issued or reissued 214 written requests for on-patent drugs, and drug sponsors declined 41 of those. FDA issued 68 written requests under BPCA for the study of on-patent drugs,[41] 20 (29 percent) of which were declined by the drug sponsors. FDA reissued 146 written requests for on-patent drugs that were originally issued under FDAMA because the pediatric drug studies had not been completed at the time BPCA went into effect. Included in the 146 were 21 (14 percent) written requests that were subsequently declined by the drug sponsors. Therefore, drug sponsors accepted 173 written requests for the study of on-patent drugs under BPCA during this period. Under FDAMA, FDA issued 227 written requests. Drug sponsors did not conduct pediatric drug studies or submit study results for 30 of the 227 (13 percent) written requests issued under FDAMA (see figure 3).[42]

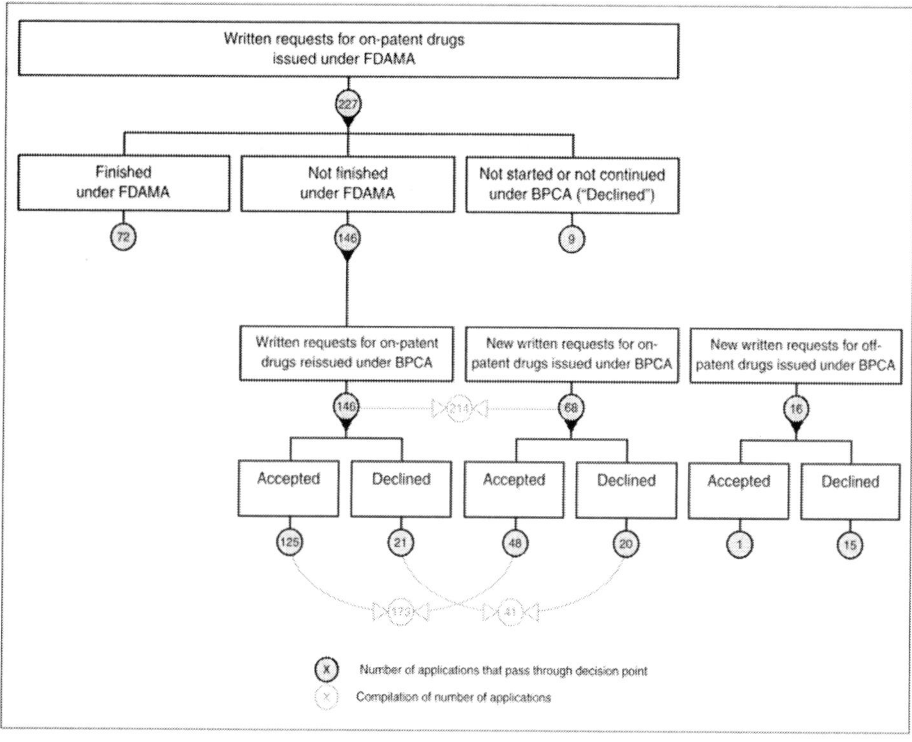

Source: GAO.

Note: If a drug sponsor of an off-patent drug does not respond to FDA's written request within 30 days, the written request is considered declined.

Figure 3. Status of Written Requests Issued under FDAMA and BPCA through December 2005

Reasons for Decline in Written Requests Issued and Accepted under BPCA Compared to FDAMA

FDA officials offered two primary reasons why fewer written requests were issued under BPCA than under FDAMA. First, according to FDA officials, when FDAMA was enacted, FDA and some drug sponsors had already identified a large number of drugs that they believed needed to be studied for pediatric use. By the time BPCA was enacted, written requests for the study of these drugs had already been issued. Second, FDA officials said there was a surge of written requests prior to the sunset of FDAMA. Agency officials expect the same surge to occur prior to the sunset of the pediatric exclusivity provisions of BPCA in 2007.

FDA officials also offered a number of reasons that the proportion of written requests issued under BPCA that were declined was greater than that for those issued under FDAMA. While FDA does not track the reasons that drug sponsors decline specific written requests, FDA officials expect that a major reason that the written requests were declined is that the agency sometimes requests more extensive pediatric drug studies, and therefore more costly studies, than the sponsors would like to do. This may be the case even when the drug sponsors initiated the written request process. FDA officials said that upon consideration of FDA's written requests, drug sponsors may make a business decision not to conduct the requested pediatric drug studies because they may be too costly for the expected return associated with pediatric exclusivity. Agency officials reported that since the drugs studied under FDAMA were more likely to be those with the greatest expected financial return or the easiest to study, they are not surprised at the higher proportion of pediatric drug studies declined under BPCA. Further, under BPCA drug sponsors are required to pay user fees—as high as $767,400 in fiscal year 2006—when study results are submitted for pediatric exclusivity consideration. As a result, the process of gaining pediatric exclusivity has become more expensive than it was under FDAMA when drug sponsors were exempt from such fees for pediatric drug studies.

FDA officials said they are not discouraged by the increase in the number of written requests that have been declined. In 2001, FDA reported to Congress that the agency expected drug sponsors to conduct pediatric drug studies for 80 percent of written requests. The rate at which written requests for studies of on-patent drugs were accepted under BPCA— 71 percent—is close to the target of 80 percent, and it is substantially larger than the 15 to 30 percent of drugs that FDA officials have reported were labeled for pediatric use prior to the authorization of pediatric exclusivity under FDAMA and BPCA.[43]

APPENDIX VI: COMPLEXITY OF COMPLETED PEDIATRIC DRUG STUDIES

The pediatric drug studies conducted under BPCA were complex and sizable, involving a large number of study sites and children. From July 2002 through December 2005,[44] drug sponsors submitted study reports to FDA in response to 59 written requests. FDA made pediatric exclusivity determinations for 55 of those written requests by December 2005, and most—51, or 93 percent—were made in 90 days or less.

For the 59 written requests for which study results were submitted to FDA, a total of 143 pediatric drug studies were conducted at 2,860 different study sites with more than 25,000 children participating (see table 7). In December 2005, FDA projected that for the drugs for which studies had not yet been submitted for review, there would be nearly 20,000 more children participating in the studies.

Table 7. Complexity of Pediatric Drug Studies Conducted under BPCA, According to Study Reports from July 2002 through December 2005

	Number of individual studies	Number of study sites for all studies	Number of participants in all studies
Count	143	2,860	25,397
Average	2	68	430
Median	2	48	255
Mode	2	83	192
Minimum	1	3	11
Maximum	7	232	2,517
Number of written req-ests data are based on	59	42	59

Source: GAO analysis of FDA data.

Appendix VII: Strengths of and Suggested Changes for BPCA

Officials from FDA and NIH discussed a number of important strengths of BPCA. In our interviews with industry group representatives and in a public forum, a number of suggestions have also been made for ways that BPCA could be improved.

Strengths of BPCA Identified by FDA and NIH Officials

FDA officials identified a number of important strengths of BCPA. Specifically, they commented on the following:

- *Economic incentives to conduct pediatric drug studies.* Because of the economic incentives in BPCA, FDA officials argue that many logistical issues inherent in conducting pediatric drug studies have been overcome. FDA may also issue a written request for pediatric drug studies for rare conditions, offering an additional incentive to develop medications for rare diseases that occur only in children.

- *Availability of summaries of pediatric drug studies.* FDA officials reported that the public dissemination of study summaries has ensured that study information is available to the health care community and has been useful to prescribers to know what has been learned about drugs' use in children.

- *Broad scope of pediatric drug studies.* BPCA allows FDA to issue written requests for pediatric drug studies for the treatment of any disease, regardless of whether the drug in question is currently indicated to treat that disease in adults. For example, FDA issued a written request for the study of a drug currently indicated to treat prostate cancer. The drug is being tested in children to see if it is effective in treating early puberty in boys.

- *Use of dispute resolution as a negotiating tool in ensuring labeling changes.* Although FDA has never invoked its authority under BPCA to use the dispute resolution process for making labeling changes, it has been an important negotiating tool. FDA officials indicated that when the agency has expressed its intention to use the process, the issues that had been raised in labeling negotiations were effectively resolved.

- *Improved safety through focused pediatric safety reviews.* BPCA's requirement that FDA conduct additional monitoring of adverse event reports for 1 year after a drug is granted pediatric exclusivity has been useful to FDA in prioritizing safety issues for children. For example, an analysis of a drug 1 year after pediatric exclusivity was granted showed that there were deaths among children as a result of overuse or misuse of the drug. This led the agency to amend the labeling regarding the appropriate population for the drug.

NIH officials said they have found the process of developing the list of drugs important for study in children to be extremely helpful. NIH officials told us that since the inception of BPCA, they have learned a great deal about existing gaps in the drug development process for children, including a lack of data about which drugs are used by children and how frequently. To gather additional information, NIH has contracted for literature reviews to decrease the possibility that unnecessary pediatric drug studies are conducted. These officials also stated that BPCA and the development of the priority list have helped to solidify an alliance between NIH and FDA, which has led to discussions and resolutions of scientific and ethical issues relating to pediatric drug studies.

Suggestions for Changes to BPCA

The Institute of Medicine convened a forum on pediatric research in June 2006 where forum participants made suggestions for how BPCA could be improved.[45] In addition, we discussed suggestions for improving BPCA with interest group representatives. Forum participants suggested that the timing of the determination of pediatric exclusivity should parallel the scientific review of a drug application and that both should be within 180 days of FDA receiving the results from the pediatric drug studies. FDA's ability to assess the overall quality of the pediatric drug studies in the 90 days currently allotted for the review was questioned. Some forum participants also stated that a longer review period could result in different determinations in some cases. For example, FDA's scientific review of data related to the study of one drug showed that the children participating in the pediatric drug studies had not received the treatments as the drug sponsors had suggested in their description of the study results. While the agency had granted the drug sponsor pediatric exclusivity based on its 90-day review to determine pediatric exclusivity, it might not have done so based on what was learned during the longer, 180-day scientific review.

In addition, it was suggested that drug sponsors be required to submit their study results for pediatric exclusivity determination at least 1 year prior to patent expiration. This would allow the generic drug industry time to better plan its release of drugs. We were told that sometimes generic drugs have had to be destroyed because pediatric exclusivity determinations were made after the generic version of the drug had been manufactured and the drug's expiration date would not allow the product to be sold.

Representatives from interest groups would like the written requests to be public information and would also like FDA to publicly announce when it receives study results that have been submitted in response to a written request. This would allow the generic drug industry to better schedule the introduction of generic drugs into the market.

Other suggestions for how the study of off-patent drugs could be more effectively encouraged were offered at the forum. A forum participant suggested that methods similar to those being adopted by the European Union be implemented. According to forum participants, under new legislation in Europe, companies that study off-patent drugs will be offered a variety of incentives, such as 10 years of data protection (meaning that the data generated to support the marketing of the drug cannot be used to support another drug, in an effort to delay competition), the right to use the existing brand name (to enable the drug sponsor to capitalize on existing brand recognition), and the ability to add a symbol to the drug labeling indicating the drug has been studied in children.

Another suggestion was that current fees paid by drug sponsors for review of their drug applications could be used to fund the study of off-patent drugs (as well as on-patent drugs that drug sponsors decline to study). These fees—$767,400 for a new drug application and $383,700 for a supplemental drug application in fiscal year 2006—are collected from drug sponsors when study results are submitted to FDA for review and consideration of pediatric exclusivity.

APPENDIX VIII: COMMENTS FROM THE DEPARTMENT OF HEALTH AND HUMAN SERVICES

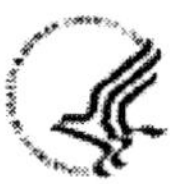

DEPARTMENT OF HEALTH & HUMAN SERVICES

Office of the Assistant Secretary for Legislation

Washington, D.C. 20201

MAR 16 2007

Ms. Marcia Crosse
Director, Health Care
U.S. Government Accountability Office
Washington, DC 20548

Dear Ms. Crosse:

Enclosed are the Department's comments on the U.S. Government Accountability Office's (GAO) draft report entitled, "Pediatric Drug Research: Studies Conducted Under Best Pharmaceuticals for Children Act" (GAO-07-557), before its publication.

We appreciate the effort that went into the analysis of Best Pharmaceuticals for Children Act statistics and information provided by FDA to GAO. We are providing General and Technical Comments on the draft report on the primary substantive issues and factual corrections. Although we had a telephone conference call with members of the GAO team on March 7, 2007, to identify factual and technical errors in the Statement of Facts provided to FDA, many of the corrections we explained to GAO on March 7 are not reflected in the draft report. To ensure the data and analysis are not subject to misinterpretation, we identify the technical corrections that should be made to the draft report.

Sincerely,

Rebecca Hemard

for Vincent J. Ventimiglia
Assistant Secretary for Legislation

Appendix VIII. (Continued)

GENERAL COMMENTS ON THE DEPARTMENT OF HEALTH AND HUMAN SERVICES ON THE GOVERNMENT ACOUNTABILITY OFFICE DRAFT REPORT ENTITLED: "PEDIATRIC DRUG RESEARCHSTUDIES CONDUCTED UNDER BEST PHARMACEUTICALS FOR CHILDREN ACT (GAO-07-557)

The HHS Food and Drug Administration (FDA) and the National Institutes of Health (NIH) are responsible for implementation of the BPCA. FDA has the primary responsibility for the BPCA exclusivity process. Although there are no recommendations on BPCA contained in the draft report for HHS *(FDA)* comment, we are providing General Comments on several key substantive issues.

While the GAO draft report has provided a significant amount of data and analysis and generally explains the BPCA process, the draft report contains several statements and characterizations, which may provide a misleading impression to Congress and other readers of the final report. We believe the general comments provided below are critical to understanding the public health benefits of BPCA and the full scope of the program as currently implemented.

- ***Success of BPCA.*** The GAO draft report does not acknowledge that BPCA is a successful program. Although the draft report includes statistics on how many drugs have been studied in pediatric populations and how many drugs have been labeled, it fails to state that the pediatric studies were conducted and drugs were labeled as a result of the BPCA process. Approximately a quarter of the products studies resulted in either new safety or dosing labeling information or information suggesting that the product was ineffective at the dose and manner in which it was studied. In addition to the important use information now in labels, BPCA has improved the infrastructure for pediatric drug development by providing additional incentives for the study of on-patent drugs, a process for the study of off-patent drugs, a vigorous and public safety review of all products granted pediatric exclusivity, and the public dissemination of information in pediatric studies conducted. As a result, BPCA has generated more clinical information for the pediatric population than any other legislative or regulatory effort to date.

  Although there have been no finished studies on certain products, such as those off-patent drugs or drugs for which the sponsor declined to conduct studies, which have gone through the NIH contracting process, these are often the most complex studies to conduct and we are confident that these efforts will show results in the next several years.

- ***Label changes under BPCA.*** The GAO draft report confuses FDA's review process for pediatric supplements with timeframes described in the BPCA for labeling dispute resolution. As written, the draft report states that it often takes a long time to make labeling changes. However, the time as reported in the draft report includes the review of the scientific data, requests for additional information, and the sponsor's submission of additional information that support any labeling changes. FDA was not negotiating labeling changes for the entire time period as reported in the draft report.

  - Pediatric studies submitted as supplements to a new drug application by sponsors in response to written requests must be treated as "priority supplements." FDA's performance goals are to review priority supplements in 180 days.

APPENDIX VIII. (CONTINUED)

GENERAL COMMENTS ON THE DEPARTMENT OF HEALTH AND HUMAN SERVICES ON THE GOVERNMENT ACOUNTABILITY OFFICE DRAFT REPORT ENTITLED: "PEDIATRIC DRUG RESEARCHSTUDIES CONDUCTED UNDER BEST PHARMACEUTICALS FOR CHILDREN ACT (GAO-07-557)

- This goal is not a BPCA mandate (although BPCA requires that pediatric supplements under BPCA receive a priority review). If FDA determines that the supplement is deficient and requests additional information from the sponsor, the first scientific review cycle is completed. A new cycle does not begin until the sponsor submits the requested information. A supplement cannot be approved and labeling negotiations generally do not begin until all of the required information from all of the review cycles is submitted and reviewed. The multiple review cycles increase the time between the initial submission and the ultimate approval of labeling change.

- If pediatric studies are submitted as a new drug application and not a supplement, then it is not required to be reviewed as a priority. FDA has a performance goal to review new drug applications in 10 months.

- If the application or supplement is otherwise ready for approval and the only outstanding issue is the need to reach agreement on labeling changes, the BPCA's dispute resolution process can be utilized. In that case, in not later than 180 days after submission of the application, the Commissioner would request that the sponsor make any labeling changes that the Commissioner deems appropriate. If the sponsor does not agree to them, the labeling issue should be referred to the Pediatric Advisory Committee. The Pediatric Advisory Committee is given 90 days after receiving such a referral to review the pediatric study reports and make a recommendation regarding appropriate labeling changes. The Commissioner then has 30 days to review the Advisory Committee recommendations and, if appropriate, make a request that the sponsor make a labeling change. If the sponsor does not agree, the Commissioner may deem the drug to be misbranded.

- ***Study of neonates under BPCA.*** The GAO draft report, in Appendix II, states that despite FDA and NIH efforts to increase inclusion of neonates, defined as children under 1 month of age, in written requests, few written requests under BPCA include neonates. BPCA requires the inclusion of neonates in pediatric studies as appropriate, but in some cases inclusion of neonates may not be appropriate for medical or ethical reasons. In addition, although no written requests have specifically required the inclusion of "neonates" as a specific group, 14 studies of 9 drugs required the inclusion of "newborns" (also defined as children under 1 month of age and which includes neonates) and 24 studies of 13 drugs required the inclusion of infants (defined as children under 4 months of age).

- ***Pediatric exclusivity attaches to an existing patent or market exclusivity.*** The GAO draft report does not mention that pediatric exclusivity under BPCA attaches to an existing listed patent or any existing marketing exclusivities held by the drug sponsor. The exclusivity is not limited to extending market exclusivity, but also attaches to existing patents even if there is no market exclusivity left on the drug in question. Like marketing exclusivity, the existence of a listed patent affects the timing of generic drug application submission and approval.

APPENDIX IX: GAO CONTACT AND STAFF ACKNOWLEDGMENTS

GAO Contact

Marcia Crosse, (202) 512-7119 or crossem@gao.gov

Acknowledgments

In addition to the contact named above, Thomas Conahan, Assistant Director; Shaunessye Curry; Cathleen Hamann; Martha Kelly; Julian Klazkin; Carolyn Feis Korman; Gloria Taylor; and Suzanne Worth made key contributions to this report.

GAO's Mission

The Government Accountability Office, the audit, evaluation and investigative arm of Congress, exists to support Congress in meeting its constitutional responsibilities and to help improve the performance and accountability of the federal government for the American people. GAO examines the use of public funds; evaluates federal programs and policies; and provides analyses, recommendations, and other assistance to help Congress make informed oversight, policy, and funding decisions. GAO's commitment to good government is reflected in its core values of accountability, integrity, and reliability.

Obtaining Copies of GAO Reports and Testimony

The fastest and easiest way to obtain copies of GAO documents at no cost is through GAO's Web site (www.gao.gov). Each weekday, GAO posts newly released reports, testimony, and correspondence on its Web site. To have GAO e-mail you a list of newly posted products every afternoon, go to www.gao.gov and select "Subscribe to Updates."

Order by Mail or Phone

The first copy of each printed report is free. Additional copies are $2 each. A check or money order should be made out to the Superintendent of Documents. GAO also accepts VISA and Mastercard. Orders for 100 or more copies mailed to a single address are discounted 25 percent. Orders should be sent to:

U.S. Government Accountability Office
441 G Street NW, Room LM
Washington, D.C. 20548

To order by Phone:	Voice:	(202)	512-6000
	TDD:	(202)	512-2537
	Fax:	(202)	512-6061

To Report Fraud, Waste, and Abuse in Federal Programs

Contact:
Web site: www.gao.gov/fraudnet/fraudnet.htm
E-mail: fraudnet@gao.gov
Automated answering system: (800) 424-5454 or (202) 512-7470

Congressional Relations

Gloria Jarmon, Managing Director, JarmonG@gao.gov (202) 512-4400 U.S. Government Accountability Office, 441 G Street NW, Room 7125 Washington, D.C. 20548

Public Affairs

Paul Anderson, Managing Director, AndersonP1@gao.gov (202) 512-4800 U.S. Government Accountability Office, 441 G Street NW, Room 7149 Washington, D.C. 20548

End Notes

[1] The drug "label" refers to written, printed, or graphic material placed on the drug container, while drug "labeling" is much broader and includes all labels and other written, printed, or graphic materials on any container, wrapper, or materials accompanying the drug. 21 U.S.C. § 321(k), (m).

[2] Provisions regarding pediatric studies of drug are generally codified at 21 U.S.C. § 355a. Pub. L. No. 107-109, 115 Stat. 1408. The market exclusivity provisions of BPCA will sunset on October 1, 2007. 21 U.S.C. § 355a(n).

[3] BPCA reauthorized and enhanced incentives for conducting pediatric drug studies that were first established in the Food and Drug Administration Modernization Act of 1997, Pub. L. No. 105-115, 111 Stat. 2296.

[4] The value of 6 months additional marketing exclusivity is difficult to assess and depends on a number of factors for which data are not available. However, a recent study estimated that for some drugs the benefit of 6 months of marketing exclusivity was quite large, while for others the return the drug sponsor received for pediatric exclusivity was less than the cost of the studies. See Jennifer S. Li, et al., "Economic Return of Clinical Trials Performed Under the Pediatric Exclusivity Program," *JAMA,* vol. 297, no. 5 (2007).

[5] FDA is an agency within the Department of Health and Human Services.

[6] Drug sponsors can obtain market exclusivity for drugs protected by patents, as well as for drugs designed to treat rare diseases, drugs consisting of new chemical entities, and already-marketed drugs approved for new uses. See for example, 21 U.S.C. §§ 355(j)(5)(F)(ii), (iii); 21 C.F.R. § 314.108 (2006). Pediatric exclusivity under BPCA attaches to an existing listed patent or any existing market exclusivity held by the drug sponsor.

[7] For purposes of this report, we refer to drugs that have patent protection or market exclusivity as on-patent and those whose patent protection or market exclusivity has ended as off-patent. This is the same terminology typically used by government agencies to describe the exclusivity status of a drug under BPCA.

[8] FDA is responsible for issuing written requests for pediatric studies, determining whether a drug merits pediatric exclusivity as a result of those studies, and all steps in between.

[9] FNIH is an independent, nonprofit corporation. The majority of funds that FNIH receives are from the private sector. Only a portion of these funds are available for FNIH to award to researchers to conduct studies related to BPCA.

[10] We previously described how FDAMA was responsible for an increase in pediatric drug studies. GAO, *Pediatric Drug Research: Substantial Increase in Studies of Drugs for Children, But Some Challenges Remain,* GAO-01-705T (Washington, D.C.: May 8, 2001).

[11] FDA generally defines the pediatric population covered under BPCA as children from birth to 16 years old, though studies have included children as old as 18. BPCA provides that neonates be included in pediatric drug studies, as appropriate. See app. II for information about federal efforts to encourage the study of drugs in neonates.

[12] FDA officials report that 51 of 134 proposed pediatric study requests submitted by drug sponsors from 2002 to 2005 did not result in written requests. Drug sponsors sometimes later submitted revised proposed pediatric study requests, which resulted in written requests.

[13] Under certain circumstances, FDA could have only 60 days to review the study report to determine pediatric exclusivity. However, FDA officials told us that under BPCA, this has never happened. Otherwise, FDA has 90 days to determine if the studies fairly respond to the written request, were conducted in accordance with commonly accepted scientific principles and protocols, and were properly submitted.

[14] Pediatric exclusivity applies to all approved uses of the drug, not just those studied in children. Therefore, if the studies find that the drug is not safe for use by children, the drug will still receive pediatric exclusivity and therefore extended market exclusivity for the adult uses of the drug.

[15] FNIH can certify that it has insufficient funds to fund the study of a drug and refer the funding to NIH.

[16] As of fiscal year 2007, NIH is required to transfer from its appropriations at least $500,000 but no more than $1.25 million to FNIH annually. This requirement was established with the enactment of the NIH Reform Act of 2006 (Pub. L. No. 109-482, 120 Stat. 3675 (2007)).

[17] The granting of pediatric exclusivity does not depend on finding that the drug is safe and effective for
pediatric use.

[18] Most drugs studied under BPCA have previously been approved for marketing in the United States, so a supplement to the original "new drug application" is submitted. If the drug studied under BPCA was not previously approved for marketing in the United States, the application would be submitted as a new drug application. FDA has a performance goal to review non-priority new drug applications in 10 months.

[19] BPCA requires that supplemental new drug applications submitted by drug sponsors be treated as "priority supplements." FDA's goal is to take action on priority supplements within 180 days.

[20] The Pediatric Advisory Committee is also responsible for reviewing reports of adverse effects related to drugs granted pediatric exclusivity after the period of exclusivity begins, among other things. The committee consists of 13 voting members, appointed by the Commissioner of FDA, who are knowledgeable in pediatric research, pediatric subspecialties, statistics, and biomedical ethics. The committee includes one representative from a pediatric health organization and one from a relevant patient or patient-family organization.

[21] Some drugs have two written requests for a variety of reasons. In some cases, FDA may have requested that the drug sponsor study the effects of the drug on different diseases. In other cases, there could be two written requests for the same drug, issued to different drug sponsors for different dosage forms of the drug. In addition, FDA told us that the specified period for studies to be completed elapsed for some written requests before the completion of studies, and the agency issued new written requests. In all of these situations, we counted each of these written requests separately. Therefore, there are more written requests than there are unique drugs with written requests.

[22] Of the 214 written requests issued by FDA, 68 were written requests first issued under BPCA. The remaining 146 written requests were originally issued under FDAMA and reissued under BPCA because drug sponsors had not responded to the written requests or completed the requested pediatric drug studies at the time that BPCA went into effect.

[23] FDA had not completed its review of the study results to determine exclusivity prior to December 2005 for the remaining four drugs.

[24] The other three drugs were denied pediatric exclusivity. The dates that drugs are granted exclusivity and also had labeling changes are available at http://www.fda.gov/cder/pediatric/labelchange.htm. The dates of exclusivity for other drugs are not available on FDA's Web site. Most of these pediatric drug studies began under FDAMA but were continued under BPCA. Most of the pediatric drug studies begun in response to written requests initially issued under BPCA have not yet been completed.

[25] When a drug sponsor of an on-patent drug declines a written request, the agency must determine if there is a continuing need for information relating to the use of the drug in children. Reasons that FDA has concluded that there is not a continuing need include the drug was not yet approved, some part of the study was being performed by the drug sponsor or another party, the drug's patent ended, the risk-benefit assessment shifted, safe alternative therapies were already on the market even though the agency had issued the written request in hope of obtaining additional valuable information, another drug may have been approved or may soon be approved with a better safety record, or there is minimal use of the drug by children.

[26] In April 2006, FNIH agreed to allocate all $4.13 million it had raised for pediatric drug studies under BPCA to fund half the cost to study one on-patent drug—baclofen. Baclofen was identified by NIH and FNIH as the highest priority on-patent drug that a drug sponsor had declined to study. NIH is responsible for developing requests for proposals for the study of on-

patent drugs for pediatric use. The requests for proposals outline the need for studies of specific drugs and include the specific details of the studies to be conducted. NIH requested proposals for the study of baclofen and has selected a contractor to perform the studies. NIH expects the cost of the study of baclofen to be about $7.8 million over 3 years, and NIH agreed to cover the costs of the study that exceed the contribution from FNIH. Because FNIH has committed all of its BPCA funds to the study of baclofen, there are no resources left for FNIH to fund the study of any other drugs.

[27] These drugs had labeling changes made after the drug sponsors submitted partial results of their studies to FDA. Because some studies were ongoing, the drug sponsors had not submitted the final study results to FDA for consideration of pediatric exclusivity.

[28] There were no off-patent drugs for which the pediatric drug studies indicated that a formulation change was necessary.

[29] These data are based on the dates on which FDA approved the labeling changes. FDA officials said that manufacturers might not immediately make approved labeling changes on the printed material associated with a marketed product. However, this information is posted on FDA's Web site, generally within 48 hours. Sponsors often update labeling on a quarterly basis or several times a year, rather than each time a labeling change is approved. FDA does not track the actual date that revised labeling enters the market. The dates that FDA agreed to these labeling changes are reported at http://www.fda.gov/cder/pediatric .

[30] National Center for Health Statistics, *2004 National Ambulatory Medical Care Survey Data File* (Hyattsville, Md.: February 2004).

[31] Medical Expenditure Panel Survey (Agency for Health Care Policy and Research, *2003 Medical Expenditure Panel Survey Household Data File* (Rockville, Md.: November 2005)).

[32] NIH is made up of 28 institutes, centers, and offices that focus on different health concerns. The mission of NIH overall is to conduct and support medical research.

[33] Pediatric pharmacology research units are primarily located in children's hospitals and academic research centers specializing in research with children.

[34] The list, published in the *Federal Register*, can include on-patent and off-patent drugs. NIH did not include on-patent drugs on this list until 2005.

[35] See 71 *Fed. Reg.* 23931-36 (Apr. 25, 2006), 70 *Fed. Reg.* 3937 (Jan. 27, 2005), 69 *Fed. Reg.* 7243-7244 (Feb. 13, 2004), 68 *Fed. Reg.* 48402 (Aug. 13, 2003), and 68 *Fed. Reg.* 2789-2790 (Jan. 21, 2003).

[36] Some drugs have two written requests; in such cases, each written request is designed to study either the effects of the drug on a different disease or dosage form, or the drug has two sponsors. In these cases, we counted each of these written requests separately. For example, Beclomethasone had written requests issued to two sponsors for different dosage forms of the drug. An additional 3 off-patent drugs were identified in 2006. From 2003 through 2006, 12 on-patent drugs have also been listed as important for study. See 71 *Fed. Reg* 23931-23936 (2006).

[37] Two of these drugs changed patent status after the off-patent written request was issued because a new formulation of each drug was approved, resulting in new patents or exclusivities. They have had new written requests issued and are now considered on-patent drugs. Both drug sponsors also declined the on-patent written requests.

[38] Since its inception, no drug has been removed from the list published in the *Federal Register,* regardless of the feasibility or likelihood of being studied.

[39] The costs reported by NIH are estimates, which may change during the course of the studies.

[40] NIH determined that these drugs were a priority for study in children and certain conditions made it appropriate to initiate studies prior to FDA being able to issue a written request.

[41] We counted all written requests individually. In some cases, FDA issued more than one written request for a drug, such as when there was more than one sponsor, when the first written request was declined by the drug sponsor and a new written request was issued when FDA became aware of new information, or when the drug was being studied for more than one disease (though these studies may also be in the same written request).

[42] Since FDAMA did not require that drug sponsors accept or decline a written request, as required by BPCA for on-patent drugs, we could not determine the exact number of written requests that were declined. Instead, we were able to determine the number of written requests for which study results were not submitted under FDAMA and the number of written requests declined when reissued under BPCA. This is the most conservative equivalent measure. FDA officials report that it is possible that studies were conducted under FDAMA and the drug sponsors decided not to submit them to FDA for exclusivity consideration.

[43] Prior to FDAMA, over a 6-year period from 1991 to 1996, only 11 of 71 requested studies were completed without such an incentive.

[44] For these analyses, we looked at study reports submitted after July 2002 because those submitted from January 2002 through June 2002 were in response to written requests issued under FDAMA, not BPCA.

[45] Forum on Drug Discovery, Development, and Translation: Addressing the Barriers to Development in Pediatrics (conference sponsored by the Institute of Medicine of the National Academies, Washington, D.C., June 2006). The program can be accessed at www.iom.edu/CMS/3740/24155/34241.aspx.

In: Safety Efforts in Pediatric Drug Development ISBN: 978-1-60741-565-7
Editor: Conor D. Byrne

Chapter 4

PEDIATRIC DRUG RESEARCH: THE STUDY AND LABELING OF DRUGS FOR PEDIATRIC USE UNDER THE BEST PHARMACEUTICALS FOR CHILDREN ACT

GAO

WHY GAO DID THIS STUDY

About two-thirds of drugs that are prescribed for children have not been studied and labeled for pediatric use, placing children at risk of being exposed to ineffective treatment or incorrect dosing. The Best Pharmaceuticals for Children Act (BPCA), enacted in 2002, encourages the manufacturers, or sponsors, of drugs that still have marketing exclusivity—that is, are on-patent—to conduct pediatric drug studies, as requested by the Food and Drug Administration (FDA). If they do so, FDA may extend for 6 months the period during which no equivalent generic drugs can be marketed. This is referred to as pediatric exclusivity. BPCA also provides for the study of off-patent drugs.

GAO was asked to testify on the study and labeling of drugs for pediatric use under BPCA. This testimony is based on *Pediatric Drug Research: Studies Conducted under Best Pharmaceuticals for Children Act,* GAO-07-557 (Mar. 22, 2007). GAO assessed (1) the extent to which pediatric drug studies were being conducted under BPCA for on-patent drugs, (2) the extent to which pediatric drug studies were being conducted under BPCA for off-patent drugs, and (3) the impact of BPCA on the labeling of drugs for pediatric use and the process by which the labeling was changed. GAO examined data about the drugs for which FDA requested studies under BPCA from 2002 through 2005 and interviewed relevant federal officials.

www.gao.gov/cgi-bin/getrpt?GAO-07-898T.

To view the full product, including the scope and methodology, click on the link above. For more information, contact Marcia Crosse at (202) 512-7119 or crossem@gao.gov.

WHAT GAO FOUND

Drug sponsors have initiated pediatric drug studies for most of the on-patent drugs for which FDA has requested such studies under BPCA, but no drugs were studied when sponsors declined these requests. Sponsors agreed to 173 of the 214 written requests for pediatric studies of on-patent drugs. In cases where drug sponsors decline to study the drugs, BPCA provides for FDA to refer the study of these drugs to the Foundation for the National Institutes of Health (FNIH), a nonprofit corporation. FNIH had not funded studies for any of the nine drugs that FDA referred as of December 2005.

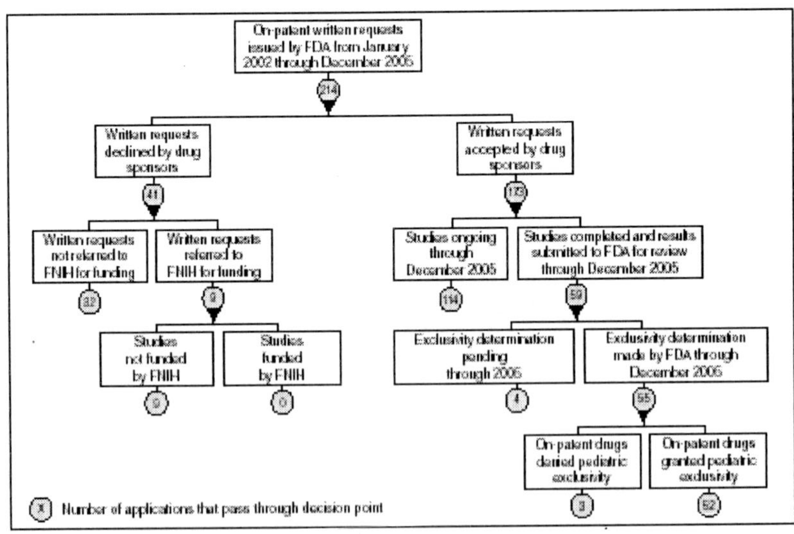

Source: GAO.

Written Requests Issued under BPCA for the Study of On-Patent Drugs (2002-2005)

Few off-patent drugs identified by the National Institutes of Health (NIH) that need to be studied for pediatric use have been studied. BPCA provides for NIH to fund studies when drug sponsors decline written requests for off-patent drugs. While 40 such off-patent drugs were identified by 2005, FDA had issued written requests for 16. One written request was accepted by the drug sponsor. Of the remaining 15, NIH funded studies for 7 through December 2005.

Most drugs granted pediatric exclusivity under BPCA (about 87 percent) had labeling changes—often because the pediatric drug studies found that children may have been exposed to ineffective drugs, ineffective dosing, overdosing, or previously unknown side effects. However, the process for approving labeling changes was often lengthy. For 18 drugs that required labeling changes (about 40 percent), it took from 238 to 1,055 days for information to be reviewed and labeling changes to be approved.

Mr. Chairman and Members of the Subcommittee:

Although children suffer from many of the same diseases as adults and are often treated with the same drugs, only about one-third of the drugs that are prescribed for children have been studied and labeled for pediatric use.[1] This has placed children taking drugs for which there have not been adequate pediatric drug studies at risk of being exposed to ineffective treatment or receiving incorrect dosing. In order to encourage the study of more drugs for pediatric use,[2] Congress passed the Best Pharmaceuticals for Children Act (BPCA) in 2002 to provide marketing incentives to drug sponsors for conducting pediatric drug studies.[3] Drug sponsors (typically drug manufacturers) may obtain 6 months of additional market exclusivity for drugs on which they have conducted pediatric studies in accordance with pertinent law and regulations.[4] This market exclusivity is known as pediatric exclusivity. When a drug has market exclusivity, it is protected from competition for a limited period; for example, the Food and Drug Administration (FDA) is prohibited from approving a generic copy for marketing.[5] Generally, pediatric exclusivity can only be granted to those drugs that are on-patent—that is, those that still have market exclusivity[6]—and for which FDA has issued a written request for pediatric drug studies.[7] However, FDA can also request pediatric drug studies for off-patent drugs—drugs for which the patent or market exclusivity has expired. BPCA also included provisions designed to provide for the study of both on-patent and off-patent drugs that drug sponsors have declined to study.

When FDA determines that a drug may provide health benefits to children, it may issue a written request to the drug sponsor to conduct pediatric drug studies on that drug. When a drug sponsor accepts a written request and conducts studies, FDA reviews the report from the pediatric drug studies to determine whether to grant pediatric exclusivity to the drug. If FDA is satisfied that the studies have been conducted and reported properly, the drug in question may receive additional market exclusivity. FDA also reviews these pediatric drug study reports to see if the drug requires labeling changes.

BPCA provides for pediatric drug studies when the drug sponsor declines the written request. First, if a drug sponsor declines a written request from FDA to study an on-patent drug, BPCA provides for FDA to refer the drug to the Foundation for the National Institutes of Health (FNIH), which can fund the study if funds are available.[8] Sponsors cannot receive pediatric exclusivity for on-patent drugs that drug sponsors decline to study. Second, BPCA provides for the funding of the study of off-patent drugs by the National Institutes of Health (NIH), which, in consultation with FDA and experts in pediatric research, identifies off-patent drugs that need to be studied for pediatric use.

My remarks today provide an overview of the study and proper labeling of drugs for pediatric use under BPCA. I will focus on (1) the extent to which pediatric drug studies were being conducted under BPCA for on-patent drugs, (2) the extent to which pediatric drug studies were being conducted under BPCA for off-patent drugs, and (3) the impact of BPCA on the labeling of drugs for pediatric use and the process by which the labeling was changed. My remarks are based upon our report assessing the effect of BPCA on pediatric drug studies and labeling.[9]

In carrying out the work for our report, we collected and analyzed a variety of data from FDA, NIH, and FNIH about written requests and pediatric studies for both on- and off-patent drugs from January 2002 through December 2005. Our work focused on actions regarding these drugs prior to 2006. To evaluate the impact of BPCA on the labeling of drugs for pediatric use and the process by which labeling was changed, we reviewed summaries of the labeling changes for drugs studied from the enactment of BPCA through 2005. In addition, to assist with our review in general, we interviewed officials from FDA, NIH, and FNIH. The work done for this statement was performed from September 2005 through March 2007 in accordance with generally accepted government auditing standards.

In summary, most of the on-patent drugs for which FDA requested pediatric drug studies under BPCA were being studied, but no studies resulted when the requests were declined by drug sponsors. Drug sponsors agreed to study 173 of the 214 on-patent drugs (81 percent) for which FDA issued written requests for pediatric drug studies from January 2002 through December 2005. Drug sponsors completed pediatric drug studies for 59 of the 173 accepted written requests—studies for the remaining 114 written requests were ongoing—and FDA made a pediatric exclusivity determination for 55 of those through December 2005. Of those 55 written requests, 52 (95 percent) resulted in FDA granting pediatric exclusivity. In addition, of the 41 on-patent drugs that drug sponsors declined to study, FDA referred 9 to FNIH, which had not funded the study of any, as of December 2005.

Few of the off-patent drugs identified by NIH as in need of study for pediatric use have been studied. By 2005, NIH had identified 40 off-patent drugs it recommended be studied for pediatric use. Through 2005, FDA issued written requests for 16 of these drugs, and all but one of these written requests were declined by drug sponsors. NIH funded pediatric drugs studies for 7 of the remaining 15 written requests declined by drug sponsors through December 2005.

Almost all the drugs that have been granted pediatric exclusivity under BPCA—about 87 percent—have had important labeling changes as a result of pediatric drug studies conducted under BPCA, but the process for reviewing the study results and making these changes can be lengthy. The labeling of drugs was often changed because the pediatric drug studies revealed that children may have been exposed to ineffective drugs, ineffective dosing, overdosing, or previously unknown side effects. The review process took from 238 to 1,055 days when FDA required additional information to support changes in the drug labeling.

BACKGROUND

BPCA was enacted on January 4, 2002, to encourage drug sponsors to conduct pediatric drug studies.[10] BPCA allows FDA to grant drug sponsors pediatric exclusivity—6 months of additional market exclusivity—in exchange for conducting and reporting on pediatric drug studies. BPCA also provides mechanisms for pediatric drug studies that drug sponsors decline to conduct.

BPCA Process

The process for initiating pediatric drug studies under BPCA formally begins when FDA issues a written request to a drug sponsor to conduct pediatric drug studies for a particular drug. When a drug sponsor accepts the written request and completes the pediatric drug studies, it submits to FDA reports describing the studies and the study results. BPCA specifies that FDA generally has 90 days to review the study reports to determine whether the pediatric drug studies met the conditions outlined in the written request.[11] If FDA determines that the pediatric drug studies conducted by the drug sponsor were responsive to the written request, it will grant a drug pediatric exclusivity regardless of the study findings.[12] Figure 1 illustrates the process under BPCA.

BPCA Provisions for Pediatric Drug Studies Declined by Drug Sponsors

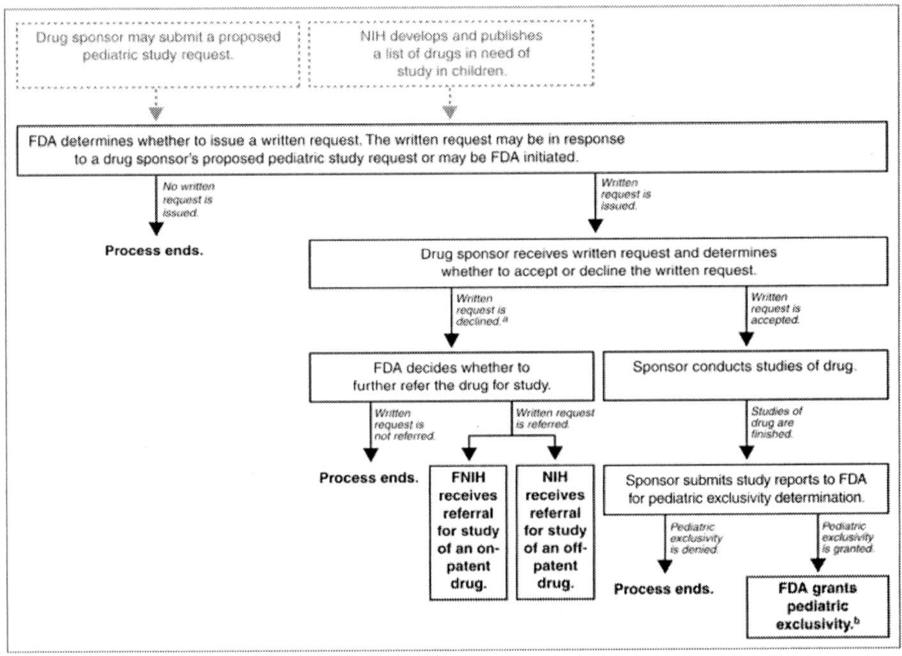

Source: GAO.

[a] If a drug sponsor of an off-patent drug does not respond to FDA's written request within 30 days, the written request is considered declined. Pediatric exclusivity is not granted to drugs where the drug sponsor declined the written request.

[b] FDA has granted pediatric exclusivity in response to written requests for on-patent drugs only. Under certain circumstances FDA could grant pediatric exclusivity in response to a written request for an off-patent drug.

Figure 1. BPCA Process

BPCA includes two provisions to further the study of drugs when drug sponsors decline written requests. FDA cannot extend pediatric exclusivity in response to written requests for any drugs for which the drug sponsors declined to conduct the requested pediatric drug studies.

First, when drug sponsors decline written requests for studies of on-patent drugs, BPCA provides for FDA to refer the study of those drugs to FNIH for funding. FNIH, which is a nonprofit corporation and independent of NIH, supports the mission of NIH and advances research by linking private sector donors and partners to NIH programs. FNIH and NIH collaborate to fund certain projects. As of December 2005, FNIH had raised $4.13 million to fund pediatric drug studies under BPCA.

Second, to further the study of off-patent drugs, NIH—in consultation with FDA and experts in pediatric research—develops a list of drugs, including off-patent drugs, which the agency believes need to be studied in children. NIH lists these drugs annually in the *Federal Register*. FDA may issue written requests for those drugs on the list that it determines to be most in need of study. If the drug sponsor declines or fails to respond to the written request, NIH can contract for, and fund, the pediatric drug studies. Drug sponsors generally decline written requests for off-patent drugs because the financial incentives are considerably limited.

Making Labeling Changes under BPCA for On-Patent Drugs

Pediatric drug studies often reveal new information about the safety or effectiveness of a drug, which could indicate the need for a change to its labeling. Generally, the labeling includes important information for health care providers, including proper uses of the drug, proper dosing, and possible adverse events that could result from taking the drug. FDA may determine that the drug is not approved for use by children, which would then be reflected in any labeling changes.

The agency refers to its review to determine the need for labeling changes as its scientific review. BPCA specifies that study results submitted as a supplemental new drug application—which, according to FDA officials, most are—are subject to FDA's general performance goals for a scientific review, which in this case is 180 days.[13] FDA's process for reviewing study results submitted under BPCA for consideration of labeling changes is not unique to BPCA. FDA's action can include approving the application, determining that the application is approvable, or determining that the application is not approvable. A determination that an application is approvable may require that drug sponsors conduct additional analyses. Each time FDA takes action on the application, a review cycle is ended.

Drug Sponsors Agreed to Study the Majority of On-Patent Drugs with Written Requests under BPCA, but No Studies Were Conducted When Drug Sponsors Declined the Written Requests

Most of the on-patent drugs for which FDA requested pediatric drug studies under BPCA were being studied, but no studies have resulted when the requests were declined by drug sponsors. From January 2002 through December 2005, FDA issued 214 written requests for on-patent drugs to be studied under BPCA, and drug sponsors agreed to conduct pediatric drug studies for 173 (81 percent) of those.[14] The remaining 41 written requests were declined. Of these 41, FDA referred 9 written requests to FNIH for funding and FNIH had not funded any of those studies as of December 2005.

Drug sponsors completed pediatric drug studies for 59 of the 173 accepted written requests—studies for the remaining 114 written requests were ongoing—and FDA made pediatric exclusivity determinations for 55 of those through December 2005.[15] Of those 55 written requests, 52 (95 percent) resulted in FDA granting pediatric exclusivity. Figure 2 shows the status of written requests issued under BPCA for the study of on-patent drugs, from January 2002 through December 2005.

Drugs were studied under BPCA for their safety and effectiveness in treating children for a wide range of diseases, including some that are common—such as asthma and allergies— and serious or life threatening in children—such as cancer, HIV, and hypertension. We found that the drugs studied under BPCA represented more than 17 broad categories of disease. The category that had the most drugs studied under BPCA was cancer, with 28 drugs. In addition, there were 26 drugs studied for neurological and psychiatric disorders, 19 for endocrine and metabolic disorders, 18 related to cardiovascular disease—including drugs related to hypertension—and 17 related to viral infections. Analyses of two national databases shows that about half of the 10 most frequently prescribed drugs for children were studied under BPCA.

Through December 2005, drug sponsors declined written requests issued under BPCA for 41 on-patent drugs. FDA referred 9 of these 41 written requests (22 percent) to FNIH for funding,[16] but as of December 2005, FNIH had not funded the study of any of these drugs.[17] NIH has estimated that the cost of studying these 9 drugs would exceed $43 million, but FNIH had raised only $4.13 million for pediatric drug studies under BPCA.

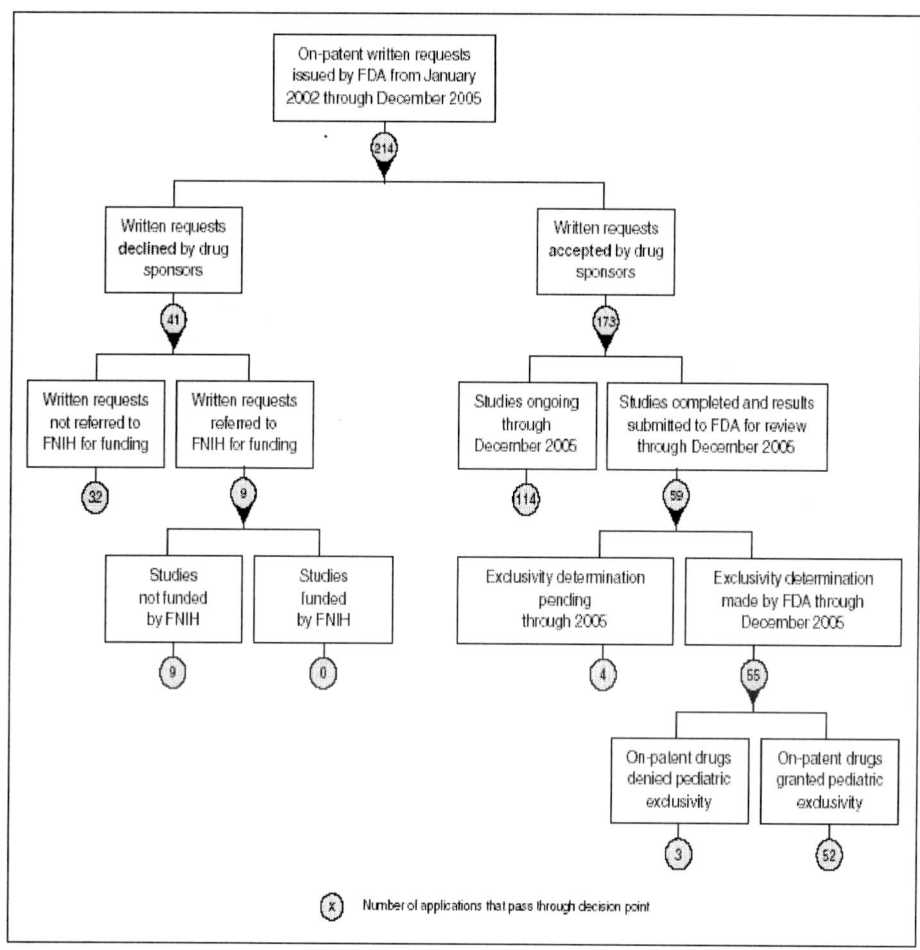

Source: GAO.

Note: Written requests issued from January 2002 through December 2005 include new written requests issued under BPCA combined with written requests originally issued under FDAMA but reissued under BPCA.

Figure 2. Status of Written Requests Issued under BPCA for the Study of On-Patent Drugs, from January 2002 through December 2005

Few Off-Patent Drugs Have Been Studied Under BPCA

Few off-patent drugs identified by NIH as in need of study for pediatric use have been studied. By 2005, NIH had identified 40 off-patent drugs that it believed should be studied for pediatric use. Through 2005, FDA issued written requests for 16 of these drugs. All but 1 of these written requests were declined by drug sponsors. NIH funded pediatric drug studies for 7 of the remaining 15 written requests declined by drug sponsors through December 2005.

NIH provided several reasons why it has not pursued the study of some off-patent drugs that drug sponsors declined to study. Concerns about the incidence of the disease that the drugs were developed to treat, the feasibility of study design, drug safety, and changes in the drugs' patent status have caused the agency to reconsider the merit of studying some of the drugs it identified as important for study in children.[18] For example, in one case NIH issued a request for proposals to study a drug but received no responses. In other cases, NIH is awaiting consultation with pediatric experts to determine the potential for study.

Further, NIH has not received appropriations specifically for funding pediatric drug studies under BPCA. NIH anticipates spending an estimated $52.5 million for pediatric drug studies associated with 7 written requests issued by FDA from January 2002 through December 2005.[19]

Most Drugs Granted Pediatric Exclusivity under BPCA Had Labeling Changes, but the Process for Making Changes Was Sometimes Lengthy

Most drugs that have been granted pediatric exclusivity under BPCA—about 87 percent—have had labeling changes as a result of the pediatric drug studies conducted under BPCA. Pediatric drug studies conducted under BPCA showed that children may have been exposed to ineffective drugs, ineffective dosing, overdosing, or side effects that were previously unknown. However, the process for reviewing study results and completing labeling changes was sometimes lengthy, particularly when FDA required additional information from drug sponsors to support the changes.

Of the 52 drugs studied and granted pediatric exclusivity under BPCA from January 2002 through December 2005, 45 (about 87 percent) had labeling changes as a result of the pediatric drug studies. In addition, 3 other drugs had labeling changes prior to FDA making a decision on granting pediatric exclusivity. FDA officials said that the pediatric drug studies conducted up to that time provided important safety information that should be reflected in the labeling without waiting until the full study results were submitted or pediatric exclusivity determined.

Pediatric drug studies conducted under BPCA have shown that the way that some drugs were being administered to children potentially exposed them to an ineffective therapy, ineffective dosing, overdosing, or previously unknown side effects—including some that affect growth and development. The labeling for these drugs was changed to reflect these study results. For example, studies of the drug Sumatriptan, which is used to treat migraines, showed that there was no benefit derived from this drug when it was used in children. There were also certain serious adverse events associated with its use in children, such as vision loss and stroke, so the labeling was changed to reflect that the drug is not recommended for children under 18 years old.

Other drugs have had labeling changes indicating that the drugs may be used safely and effectively by children in certain dosages or forms. Typically, this resulted in the drug labeling being changed to indicate that the drug was approved for use by children younger than those for whom it had previously been approved. In other cases, the changes reflected a new formulation of a drug, such as a syrup that was developed for pediatric use, or new directions for preparing the drug for pediatric use were identified in the pediatric drug studies conducted under BPCA.

Although FDA generally completed its first scientific review of study results—including consideration of labeling changes—within its 180-day goal, the process for completing the review, including obtaining sufficient information to support and approve labeling changes, sometimes took longer. For the 45 drugs granted pediatric exclusivity that had labeling changes, it took an average of almost 9 months after study results were first submitted to FDA for the sponsor to submit and the agency to review all of the information it required and approve labeling changes. For 13 drugs (about 29 percent), FDA completed this scientific review process and approved labeling changes within 180 days. It took from 181 to 187 days for the scientific review process to be completed and labeling changes to be approved for 14 drugs (about 31 percent). For the remaining 18 drugs (about 40 percent), FDA took from 238 to 1,055 days to complete the scientific review process and approve labeling changes. For 7 of those drugs, it took more than a year to complete the scientific review process and approve labeling changes.

While the first scientific reviews were generally completed within 180 days, it took 238 days or more for 18 drugs.[20] For those 18 drugs, FDA determined that it needed additional information from the drug sponsors in order to be able to approve the drugs for pediatric use. This often required that the drug sponsor conduct additional analyses or pediatric drug studies. FDA officials said they could not approve any changes to drug labeling until the drug sponsor provided this information. Drug sponsors sometimes took as long as 1 year to gather the additional necessary data and respond to FDA's request.[21]

Mr. Chairman, this concludes my prepared remarks. I would be pleased to respond to any questions that you or other members of the Subcommittee may have.

For further information regarding this testimony, please contact Marcia Crosse at (202) 512-7119 or crossem@gao.gov. Contact points for our Offices of Congressional Relations and Public Affairs may be found on the last page of this testimony. Thomas Conahan, Assistant Director; Carolyn Feis Korman; and Cathleen Hamann made key contributions to this statement.

GAO's Mission

The Government Accountability Office, the audit, evaluation and investigative arm of Congress, exists to support Congress in meeting its constitutional responsibilities and to help improve the performance and accountability of the federal government for the American people. GAO examines the use of public funds; evaluates federal programs and policies; and provides analyses, recommendations, and other assistance to help Congress make informed oversight, policy, and funding decisions. GAO's commitment to good government is reflected in its core values of accountability, integrity, and reliability.

Obtaining Copies of GAO Reports and Testimony

The fastest and easiest way to obtain copies of GAO documents at no cost is through GAO's Web site (www.gao.gov). Each weekday, GAO posts newly released reports, testimony, and correspondence on its Web site. To have GAO e-mail you a list of newly posted products every afternoon, go to www.gao.gov and select "Subscribe to Updates."

Order by Mail or Phone

The first copy of each printed report is free. Additional copies are $2 each. A check or money order should be made out to the Superintendent of Documents. GAO also accepts VISA and Mastercard. Orders for 100 or more copies mailed to a single address are discounted 25 percent. Orders should be sent to:

U.S. Government Accountability Office
441 G Street NW, Room LM
Washington, D.C. 20548

To order by Phone:	Voice:	(202)	512-6000
	TDD:	(202)	512-2537
	Fax:	(202)	512-6061

To Report Fraud, Waste, and Abuse in Federal Programs

Contact:
Web site: www.gao.gov/fraudnet/fraudnet.htm
E-mail: fraudnet@gao.gov
Automated answering system: (800) 424-5454 or (202) 512-7470

Congressional Relations

Gloria Jarmon, Managing Director, JarmonG@gao.gov (202) 512-4400 U.S. Government Accountability Office, 441 G Street NW, Room 7125 Washington, D.C. 20548

PUBLIC AFFAIRS

Paul Anderson, Managing Director, AndersonP1@gao.gov (202) 512-4800 U.S. Government Accountability Office, 441 G Street NW, Room 7149 Washington, D.C. 20548

End Notes

[1] The drug "label" refers to written, printed, or graphic material placed on the drug container while drug "labeling" is much broader and includes all labels and other written, printed, or graphic materials on any container, wrapper, or materials accompanying the drug. 21 U.S.C. § 321(k), (m).

[2] FDA generally defines the pediatric population covered under BPCA as children from birth to 16 years old, though studies have included children as old as 18.

[3] Provisions regarding pediatric studies of drugs are generally codified at 21 U.S.C. § 355a. Pub. L. No. 107-109, 115 Stat. 1408. The market exclusivity provisions of BPCA will sunset on October 1, 2007.

[4] The value of 6 months additional marketing exclusivity is difficult to assess and depends on a number of factors for which data are not available. However, a recent study estimated that for some drugs, the benefit of 6 months of marketing exclusivity was quite large, while for others the return the drug sponsor received for pediatric exclusivity was less than the cost of the studies. See Jennifer S. Li, et al., "Economic Return of Clinical Trials Performed Under the Pediatric Exclusivity Program," *JAMA*, vol. 297, no. 5 (2007).

[5] Drug sponsors can obtain additional market exclusivity or patent protection for drugs protected by patents, drugs designed to treat rare diseases, drugs consisting of new chemical entities, and already-marketed drugs approved for new uses. *See, for example,* 21 U.S.C. §§ 355(j)(5)(F)(ii), (iii); 21 C.F.R. § 314.108 (2006). Pediatric exclusivity under BPCA attaches to an existing listed patent or any existing market exclusivity held by the drug sponsor.

[6] For purposes of this statement, we refer to drugs that have patent protection or market exclusivity as on-patent and those whose patent protection or marketing exclusivity has ended as off-patent. This is the same terminology typically used by government agencies to describe the exclusivity status of a drug under BPCA.

[7] FDA is responsible for issuing written requests for pediatric studies, determining whether a drug merits pediatric exclusivity as a result of those studies, and all steps in between.

[8] FNIH is an independent, nonprofit corporation. The majority of funds that FNIH receives are from the private sector. Only a portion of these funds are available for FNIH to award to researchers to conduct studies related to BPCA.

[9] GAO, Pediatric Drug Research: Studies Conducted under Best Pharmaceuticals for Children Act, GAO-07-557 (Washington, D.C.: Mar. 22, 2007).

[10] BPCA reauthorized and enhanced the pediatric exclusivity provisions of the Food and Drug Administration Modernization Act of 1997 (FDAMA), Pub. L. No. 105-115, 111 Stat. 2296, which first established incentives for conducting pediatric drug studies—in the form of additional market exclusivity—and whose pediatric exclusivity provisions expired on January 1, 2002. We previously described how FDAMA was responsible for an increase in pediatric drug studies. GAO, *Pediatric Drug Research: Substantial Increase in Studies of Drug for Children, But Some Challenges Remain*, GAO-01-705T (Washington, D.C.: May 8, 2001).

[11] Under certain circumstances, FDA could have only 60 days to review the study report to determine pediatric exclusivity. However, FDA officials told us that under BPCA, this has never

happened. Otherwise, FDA has 90 days to determine if the studies fairly respond to the written request, were conducted in accordance with commonly accepted scientific principles and protocols, and were properly submitted.

[12] Pediatric exclusivity applies to all approved uses of the drug, not just those studied in children. Therefore, if the studies find that the drug is not safe for use by children, the drug will still receive pediatric exclusivity and therefore extended market exclusivity for the adult uses of the drug.

[13] Most drugs studied under BPCA have previously been approved for marketing in the United States, so a supplement to the original "new drug application" is submitted. BPCA requires that supplemental new drug applications submitted by drug sponsors be treated as "priority supplements." FDA's goal is to take action on priority supplements within 180 days. If the drug studied under BPCA was not previously approved for marketing in the United States, the application would be submitted as a new drug application. FDA has a performance goal to review nonpriority new drug applications in 10 months.

[14] Some drugs have two written requests for a variety of reasons. In some cases, FDA may have requested that the drug sponsor study the effects of the drug on different diseases. In other cases, there could be two written requests for the same drug, issued to different drug sponsors for different dosage forms of the drug. In addition, FDA told us that the specified time period for studies to be completed elapsed for some written requests before the completion of studies, and the agency issued new written requests. In all of these situations, we counted each of these written requests separately. Therefore, there are more written requests than there are unique drugs with written requests. Of the 214 written requests issued by FDA, 68 were written requests first issued under BPCA. The remaining 146 written requests were originally issued under FDAMA and reissued under BPCA because drug sponsors had not responded to the written requests or completed the requested pediatric drug studies at the time that BPCA went into effect.

[15] FDA had not completed its review of the study results to determine exclusivity prior to December 2005 for the remaining four drugs.

[16] When a drug sponsor of an on-patent drug declines a written request, the agency must determine if there is a continuing need for information relating to the use of the drug in children. Reasons that FDA has concluded that there is not a continuing need include the drug was not yet approved, some part of the study was being performed by the drug sponsor or another party, the drug's patent ended, the risk-benefit assessment shifted, safe alternative therapies were already on the market even though the agency had issued the written request in hope of obtaining additional valuable information, another drug may have been approved or may soon be approved with a better safety record, or there is minimal use of the drug by children.

[17] In April 2006, FNIH agreed to allocate all $4.13 million it had raised for pediatric drug studies under BPCA to fund half of the cost to study one on-patent day—baclofen. NIH expects the cost of the study of baclofen to be about $7.8 million over three years and NIH agreed to cover the costs of the study that exceed the contribution from FNIH. Because FNIH has committed all of its BPCA funds to the study of baclofen, there are no resources left for FNIH to fund the study of any other drugs.

[18] Since its inception, no drug has been removed from the list published in the *Federal Register*, regardless of the feasibility or likelihood of it being studied.

[19] The costs reported by NIH are estimates, which may change during the course of the studies.

[20] FDA considers itself in conformance with its review goals even though the entire process often took longer than 180 days.

[21] BPCA provides a dispute resolution process that FDA can use to resolve disagreements with drug sponsors regarding labeling of on-patent drugs where the only remaining issue concerns the labeling. FDA officials said they have never used this process because labeling has never been the only unresolved issue for those drugs for which the review period exceeded 180 days. Agency officials told us that reminding the drug sponsors that such a process exists has

motivated drug sponsors to complete labeling change negotiations by reaching agreement with FDA.

INDEX

A

B

C

D

E

F

G

H

I

J

K

L

M

N

O

P

R

S

T

U

V

W

Y